MW00480104

THE FIFTH
EPISODE

INSIDE THE MANIC MIND

GARRETT CAMPBELL

THE FIFTH EPISODE

INSIDE THE MANIC MIND

Garrett Campbell

ISBN (Print Edition): 978-1-66784-345-2

ISBN (eBook Edition): 978-1-66784-346-9

CONTENTS

EPISODE 1

THE SUN, MY MOST BRILLIANT CREATION, WAS SHINING perfectly. The water was calm. She was beautiful beyond all measure. We had done it. We would change the world and we would do it with the power of love. It was my only focus. Nothing else mattered. Not money. Not my past. I had only to live in the moment and follow the instructions being placed in my mind from a higher power. I realized that my thoughts were different, but they were better. They were addictive. I wanted more. How high would he allow me to level up? In my mind, I was already an *infinite level human.*

I thought to myself, "If I can stay up for another couple nights without sleeping, he might give me the answers I desire. I must prove to him that I am worthy." It shouldn't be hard now that I have an open line of communication with him. I looked around at my surroundings. "I can't believe I've had all this my whole life and didn't realize it." I was sitting on a small beach in front of my bungalow in Big Pond, Nova Scotia. I had the girl of my dreams by my side and, in this moment, it didn't matter we were only dating for months – I wanted to marry her.

We had old ripped towels underneath us, but they were perfect; they were just what we needed. A bottle of Nova 7 and Avondale Sky Bliss rested by our sides next to a bowl of grapes. It was finally time to live like a God. Many goals had been accomplished in the nights leading to this moment, but I knew I was only scratching the surface. "Hannah, pour some bliss into my mouth and feed me some grapes," I said with confidence. "Ok, babe," she muttered. After she fulfilled my request, I thought she deserved to enjoy herself. I was saddened that she had not yet leveled up to a higher dimensional being like myself, but I knew that I could show her the way if she allowed me to do my work. I grabbed the wine and told her to open her mouth. She enjoyed the taste of the wine and the grapes that followed. I decided at that moment I would treat her like a goddess for the rest of time. It would be Hannah and me – forever; we would travel the universe together.

I could feel my brain pulsate in the back of my head. Another message was coming. Did I finally do it? Did I prove to God I understand the secrets of the universe? Was he going to bring us to him to meet? I stood up with the wine, tilted my head back and poured myself a mouthful - calm with perfect precision. My confidence was unworldly. As I slowly lowered my head and gazed upon the glass-like lake, I noticed something out of the corner of my left eye. I turned my head with a sense of optimism. My optimism quickly turned into anxiety.

They were coming for me. They knew my power was too great. I couldn't be left alone. Four Cape Breton Regional Police Officers were slowly walking towards me from the direction of my family compound. Their hats were off. Their gloves were worn. They were walking two by two. I quickly scanned them – Four pistols on their sides. I knew I had only a moment to make a decision before they made their way to Hannah and I. My sandals were lying next to me on the rocky shore. First, I thought of taking control. I could bend down to grab my sandals as they approached, rise up with a stone and take out the largest man. The rest should be taken back momentarily. This will give me enough time for one more swing; I'll target the man in the front left. Only two remaining. I know they'll go for their guns. I'll aim for the throat of the man in the back wearing red hair. He looks weak. Then it will be one on one; I'd always bet on myself. With my newly found abilities granted from God, they wouldn't stand a chance. I could then finish them with the first stone.

My brain pulsated again, this time more near the crown of my head. It was as if I was flexing my brain. It was painful. Was this the cost of the open line of communication with my fellow infinites? I turned to Hannah. "It's ok, Garrett," she said with sympathy. In what felt like a millisecond, I thought of a new plan. I would grab Hannah by the hand, run up the ten-foot embankment, and enter the woods. I would use my military training to navigate through the woods to the highway and we would flag down a car. I had to get her out of here. I turned to the officers. They were now close enough to say their first words.

"Are you Garrett Campbell? We just want to talk," said the largest officer in a calming voice. So many thoughts flashed through my mind. How can this be happening? I was so close. I was almost there. A god on Earth. The god of love. I dropped to my knees. I offered my hands to be cuffed. I was devastated. "You're not under arrest, Garrett. We just want to talk to you; your family is concerned." I stood up, took a deep breath, and locked my eyes on the first officer. I stared into his eyes briefly. Then into the eyes of the next officer. Then the next. And finally, the fourth. I decided to cooperate.

I couldn't get myself to look back at Hannah. I felt like a failure. I was going to give her the universe, and now it was all over. The worst part of it all was that my family, the ones I love the most, were the reason I failed. Perhaps I shouldn't have shared my secrets with them. Maybe I should have kept my newly found skills to myself and been more selfish. I can't do this, though. I need everyone to know of my new wisdom and level up to an infinite with me. It's the only way to save humans.

We finally started up the beach towards my cottage. We were walking with two police officers in the front, two in the back, and me in the middle. Hannah was trailing behind. The towels, grapes, and wine stayed at our spot on the beach. I remember how badly I wanted to stay in our spot and finish our day together. The pain was unbearable. It was my chance to finally relax after getting so much done.

As we turned the corner and the compound opened. All my family were standing there watching me. I was the main attraction. There were two police cars, an ambulance with two paramedics, aunts, uncles, family, and first cousins. All eyes were on me. The police sat me down on a bench by the fire pit near the beach. "What's going on, Garrett?" the policeman said with a look of concern over his face. I could feel the anxiety taking over; my heart was pounding. I rambled, "Listen to me. Some of my friends and I have been working with a network marketing company, and we've been killing it! We broke some of the Canadian records for sales in just the first couple days. We're only getting started. We decided to make a group called Elite 8 Lifestyle because we're going to be making so much money that we have a huge opportunity to donate money to charity. That's what it means to be elite. You make money, but then you donate it to help make people feel loved. We're going to solve everyone's problems with love!"

The cop replied, "Listen, Garrett, your family is really concerned with the way you've been acting lately. Would you consider going to the hospital to be checked out?"

"You're not listening to me! Don't you understand?" I shouted back as my eyes widened.

He responded, "Garrett, I know you're really excited and you want to do a good thing here, but I can tell that you're really stressed. Don't you think it would be good to talk to a doctor and make sure you're doing alright?"

"I don't need a doctor! My family is concerned because I haven't been sleeping. They don't get it. That's how you get things done! At basic training, I stayed up for four days straight during the final exercises! When I told my family about that, they said it was amazing! Now I stay up for a couple of days and it's like the world is ending!" I was speaking rapidly with heavy emotion. I was ready to break down into tears. All I could think about was the great things I wanted to achieve and how close I was to success. I felt like everyone I loved was against me. No one understood that I was trying to save them all.

The cop responded, "Garrett. It's ok. I can tell you're hurting right now. I was a military man myself. I served with the military police. You can trust me, man."

"Then let's donate one million fucking dollars to the Soldier On program! You can come on stage with me to present the check. We'll gather all the top military officers from around Canada. It will be perfect," I said with complete desperation.

Just as the officer was opening his mouth to reply, I could hear the large officer shout from behind the benches. He was standing with the other policemen and the paramedics. "Alright, let's wrap this up! We can't be tying up all of these resources any longer." As he finished, I could see my first cousin, Elijah, walk over to him with purpose. They whispered to each other for what felt like an eternity but was most likely only seconds. They turned and started towards me. As they approached, the large officer, who I could now tell was the captain, told me what was going to happen. "Alright, Garrett, we're going to have to take you to the hospital. Your cousin here had the idea that they would take you in, so you don't have to travel in the back of a patrol car. Does that sound good to you?" I wanted to cry; however, I knew my purpose was too great to show weakness. I replied, "Ok." I was fighting off the tears with everything I had left. I suddenly felt tired for the first time in days, but my energy was still high. It was the ultimate form of exhaustion.

"Can I get a shirt before we go?" I requested. I was only wearing a bathing suit and sandals. They agreed begrudgingly, and we headed over to my cottage. As we made our way over, I walked by the crowd consisting of over fifteen family members. I had a feeling of embarrassment. I felt angry. I felt sad. Every possible emotion was rushing through my mind. My brain hurt again. I kept my chin high. I needed to figure out how to cooperate but still be able to complete my mission. There were only two policemen escorting me this time. They must have realized that I wasn't a violent person despite what my family must have told them upon arrival. I remember thinking as I walked into the cottage I didn't notice my father in the crowd. I knew he was there in the morning when we got up. Where was he now?

"Hurry up, Garrett. We have to go." The officers rushed me onward. I went down through the cluttered hallway into my bedroom that consisted of a dresser and a mattress and box spring stacked on the floor. The doorway to the room was a curtain hanging on a rod. It was set up in a way that anything said in the bedroom could be heard in neighboring rooms. I opened a drawer of the dresser and looked through my shirts. After flipping through two or three, one officer grabbed a shirt off the floor and told me to put it on. I agreed. I exited my bedroom, walked back through the hallway and into the main living space where the kitchen on the left was open to the living area on the right. I paused as I noticed the kitchen table; $750 worth of liquor sitting on the tablet laid out as a display for the pictures taken the night before. I remembered the curiosity it spiked when we posted those pictures to social media. I smiled and I relinquished in the fact that I figured out social media marketing in just one night. My skills were impressive.

"Garrett. Let's go." I could sense frustration building in the voice of the officer. I turned my head from the table and made my way out the patio doors and onto the deck. I took a left towards the steps and the crowd. Everyone was still in place, but one of the police cars was gone as well as ambulance. I had to walk by my family one last time. My sister approached me, "Listen, Elijah and I are going to take you in his truck, and the police are going to follow us in to make sure everything goes smoothly." I appreciated not having to travel by police cruiser, but I couldn't get past the rage building inside, knowing that my family was trying to stop me from achieving my goals. They were conspiring against me.

As I hoped into the back of the truck, I took my phone out of my side pocket; the police didn't notice I grabbed it while I was in my bedroom looking for a shirt. I instantly sent a text message to my friend Noah. He had slept at my cottage the night before and left earlier that morning to find new preferred clients and consultants for our business. "Noah, my family called the police on me. I'm on my way to the hospital. This is crazy." I assumed I would get an instant reply, but it never came. He was as energetic about the business as I was and as full of belief. We both knew we had something special. It was only a matter of time before the world saw it unfold.

Elijah and my sister, Melissa, tried to make conversation on the drive into Sydney, but I would shrug off their questions replying with a quick yes, no, or uh-huh. I had only thirty minutes before arriving at the hospital, and I had to make the most of it. I switched over from my messaging app to Twitter. I had to make sure #elite8lifestyle was still trending. My friends and I had put out hundreds of tweets the night before simultaneously to take the world by storm. We would not take any chances. We needed it to trend so we could spread love across the globe. Typing in just a few characters, I saw it appear. In my mind, it was still spreading. I texted Noah to let him know our plan was working. Still no response.

As we passed by Big Pond beach, I looked down, and I could remember taking swimming lessons as a child. All my cousins would show up together and wait for our instructor. Some mornings were so cold we would stay in our clothing until the very last possible second. Other mornings we would show up early if the weather was good and horse around in the water before classes would start. I remember thinking to myself that I missed those days. I loved my cousins so much, and the thought of them betraying me brought on a pain I've never felt before. How could things have changed so much they thought I was sick just because I wanted to spread love across the world? They must have misunderstood me. They must not have known that my intentions were pure. I was doing this for them, the people I loved most.

On the other side of the street was the Big Pond Church. We used to attend mass there as children. As I gazed upon it, I could feel my sadness turn into a strong sense of power and purpose. I felt as though I needed to visit the church and speak with the priest. He would understand me. He would believe that I am a god walking amongst men. I knew I couldn't tell my family, but a man of faith would understand me. I made a mental note to return to the church at my earliest convenience, for it was my home.

During the next twenty minutes of the drive, I realized that each car to pass by us knew of my situation. They knew that I was trying to change the world for the better, but they wouldn't stop to help me; they drove by as if nothing was going on. I tried to lock eyes with each driver because I felt it was wrong for me not to acknowledge them. How could they pass by and continue with their day, knowing that such a powerful being was just feet away from them? I checked Twitter again – still trending. My power level grew. Was it possible? Was there another level I could reach?

Then I saw it. Just over the trees on the left side of the highway, I could see the roof of the Cape Breton Regional Hospital. I calculated that we would arrive in three minutes. I zoned in, trying to be present. I could convince them. I knew I had to level back down to a basic human form so I wouldn't be misunderstood. I needed them to know I was ok so they would let me go back to my cottage and fulfil my duty as a god on Earth. I had to do this for the infinites in the universe. This was much bigger than me. The universe hung in the balance. If I messed this up, it would all be over. Everyone I love would never know the true meaning of life as I do.

As we pulled up to the hospital, my anxiety rose as did my confidence to match it. I wasn't scared of this place. I was scared to deal with humans on a vibration lower than myself. My frequency was vibrating at a level that no one in this building could understand. No one in this world could understand. My only fear was that they would fear me and not understand that I only wanted to help them.

We entered the emergency room, and I sat down at triage in my wrinkly shirt, dirty bathing suit, and sandals. "Put this under your tongue," said the nurse as she placed a thermometer in my mouth. "Lift your arm," she commanded. She placed a blood pressure cuff over my arm and a heart rate monitor on my finger. I knew, in this moment, she was dying to see the results. It was more than likely the first time she's taken vitals of an infinite – of a god. After she was done, I made my way back into the waiting room but only for a moment. They were quick to get me into a private room. I assumed it was for my own protection. There were too many low-level beings in the waiting room. It wasn't safe for me there.

I was in the treatment room for a moment by myself. I had to act quickly. I grabbed my phone and took a picture of the room. I captured enough of the equipment so my location would be obvious to anyone who saw the photo. I opened Twitter, attached the photo, and captioned it "Thanks everyone #elite8lifestyle." I knew someone would see it and come rescue me. It would at least signal to my team that I've been taken in so they would know to continue with the mission without me and come see me if need be.

When Melissa and Elijah entered the room to wait with me, I was furious. Despite my disappointment in them and my general anger, I made one last attempt to reverse the situation. "Guys, this is all a misunderstanding. Look, I have a friend that works with me at the base in Halifax. His name is Brad. He's awesome. He's from Antigua. He told me if I ever wanted to go visit him while he's there, it wouldn't be a problem. Let's just put this behind us and get out of here. Let's go to Antigua. I know you guys don't have the money for a trip right now, but don't worry about it – I'll pay for all of us!"

They looked at each other for a moment and turned back to me. "Garrett, we think it would be best for you to talk to the doctor first, then we can discuss whatever you'd like." My irritability rapidly grew. "Why don't you believe in me? I love you guys and I'm just trying to help you!" I said with desperation. My heart was broken. I couldn't come to terms with everyone being seemingly against me. I knew deep down I had to stay strong, but my frustration was building up and I could feel my thoughts race. I tried to focus on my mission. I was the only person who had the power to save humans. How could I do what needed to be done while I was stuck in a hospital? My only choice was to try and convince the doctor that what I was doing to right. I had to make them see things my way. Surely, they would understand.

I laid on the observation table for what seemed like an eternity. Changing my position every minute or so. Sitting up, laying down, and tossing from side to side. I couldn't stay still. Eventually, the door opened, and a doctor finally entered the room. "Hi, Garrett, my name is Dr. MacDonald. I'm a resident here at the Regional. Can we chat?" I sat up with my back straight and said in what I felt was a calm voice, "sure." He asked me, "So what's been going on lately? Your family is concerned that you've been acting a little different than your regular self the last couple of days. I understand that you started a new business?"

I replied, "Yes, I'm glad you brought that up. A few friends and I started to work with a network marketing company, and we've been killing it! We been breaking records and building a strong team! My family doesn't understand how it works so they're trying to stop us. They think it's a scam. I tried to explain it to them, but they just won't listen. They don't believe in me! They won't accept that I'm doing it for them!"

The rest of the conversation is a blur. I can't quite recall the follow-up questions, but we talked for about 10 to 15 minutes before he told me I would have to provide a urine sample. My initial thought was that they knew of my newly realized abilities, and they wanted to test my urine to see how its composition differed from that of a normal human. Then it hit me. I recalled that for that last few nights, I've been smoking cannabis. If they test my urine and cannabis comes up in the screening, they would notify the military and I would be released from service.

The small part of my intact mind that remained thought of all my goals in life. I was proud to be a member of the Canadian forces. I admittedly joined for the wrong reasons, but once I got to basic training, I knew it was for me. I excelled in every aspect of the fifteen-week training. My final candidate score was ten out of ten and I even was awarded top athlete of my platoon. People there looked up to me. They would praise my fitness and ask for advice on how they can improve. I made lifelong friends and looked forward to going to work. It was the perfect fit for me - a great balance of work and physical training.

There was also an opportunity to travel the world playing Basketball, which was a dream come true. I joined the CFB Halifax base team shortly after basic training, and after capturing the team's tenth consecutive Regional Championship, we travelled to Ontario to compete in Nationals. After a hard-fought tournament, we narrowly edged out the win in the finals and won the first National title for CFB Halifax. I was picked up during the tournament to try out for the Canadian Forces CISM National team and eventually travelled to Brazil to compete in the Military World Games in Rio de Janerio. I remember thinking so often during that time in my life how perfect my life was. I had everything I would ever need.

I couldn't let this doctor take it all away from me. It was ok though, I had plan. He handed me the clear cup with an orange lid. He pointed out a line to me. "Just fill it up to here," he said. I told him, "Just so you know, I've been drinking a lot of dissolving vitamin tablets the last couple of days, so this is going to be pretty yellow. It might even be green." He laughed and said, "That's okay, Garrett. Go ahead and fill it up." He closed the door as his laugh trailed off. It was time to put my plan into action. I knew this would be the hardest thing I've done to date. I had to push myself and really test out my newly found abilities. I undid my shorts and let them drop to my ankles. I held my shirt under my chin, unscrewed the lid and held the cup in place over the toilet. I was ready.

I closed my eyes and placed my free hand on my abdomen. I focused on my kidneys. I knew that the only way out of this situation was to have my kidneys filter out the cannabis from my urine. I had to command my body to keep the cannabis in my bloodstream. If any got through, I would lose everything. I took a deep breath and opened my eyes as wide as humanly possible. I began to urinate. I was flexing what I thought to be my brain to where my head vibrated and I thought to myself, "It's working."

I placed the cup on the rim of the toilet, pulled up my shorts, and tied them. I bent down towards the toilet and grabbed the cup. I had filled it over the line, so I poured out some urine ever so slowly. It had to be perfect. After being satisfied with the volume level, I grabbed some toilet paper and cleaned around the rim of the cup. "That looks good," I thought. I sealed the lid and stood up. One last check. I held the cup up to my eyes and stared into it with laser focus. I was analyzing the particles inside of the urine. No cannabis.

Satisfied with my work, I opened the door and handed the cup to the intern. "See, I told you it was going to be yellow." He chuckled, took the cup, and led me back to the treatment room. Just as I was approaching the doorway, I could see to my left that Melissa and Elijah were talking to an African American man dressed like a businessman. He was wearing nice brown dress shoes, black dress pants, a white button-up top, and a dark grey blazer. I assumed he was sent to help me. Maybe I wasn't the only god in Cape Breton. Maybe there are others out there who want to help me. Surely, if they know what I know, they would help me gain my freedom.

I entered the treatment room and hopped back up onto the observation table. Every minute felt like ten as my irritability was still running high. I remember thinking how curious I was to see the look on the lab technician's face when they realized that the urine, they were testing wasn't that of a normal human. I smiled to myself and laughed under my breath. My enjoyment was interrupted as Melissa entered the room. "Hey, Garrett, we were just talking with a psychiatrist, and he's going to come chat with you, ok?" I couldn't believe what I just heard. A psychiatrist? My sister thought I was crazy. After all of the work I had put in over the last month, it's going to be played off as if I've lost my mind. The anger I felt at that moment was unlike anything I've ever experienced. "Whatever, Melissa!" I replied.

It felt like the walls were closing in on me. I could feel my heart rate rising and my breaths shortening. "So, this is how they do it…" I thought to myself. Whenever they find someone like me who realizes their true potential, they make them out to seem crazy. Thoughts were flowing through my mind at a rate I hadn't yet experienced. For the first time, I couldn't think of a way out. I couldn't solve the problem. I felt defeated.

The psychiatrist entered the room, introduced himself and sat down. "So, Garrett, I understand you've been working on a new business recently. Can you tell me a bit about that?" "Yes. I joined a network marketing company and I've been killing it. I broke a bunch of records for sales in the first month. Some of my friends joined with me and we're doing it together." The tone in my voice was filled with arrogance and irritation.

"What is Elite8Lifestlye?" he asked. "Elite8Lifestyle is the name of our group. It's eight people that want to use what we're doing to change the lives of the people we love. Is that bad or is it ok to love people and want to help them?" My eyes were widening as I responded. I was staring right into the eyes of the psychiatrist. I continued. "Look, all we're doing is trying to capture the good in the world and put it out there on Twitter. We see something that we love, and we post it. Love is infectious and people will be inspired by it!"

The psychiatrist paused. "Why are you posting pictures of your family on Twitter?"

"BECAUSE I LOVE THEM!" I yelled.

Then he said it. The first time I would hear this word as being a part of my life. The word that would haunt me annually for the next five years. "Garrett, you are experiencing mania right now, and we are going to have to admit you to the ward." He stood up and exited the room. I wanted to cry, but I could show no signs of weakness. I still don't know if my brain truly would allow me to feel sadness or if I tricked myself into thinking it was an opportunity to show my family they couldn't break me.

Hannah and Melissa entered the room shortly after and asked me how I felt. I tried to make my case to them one last time. I tried to explain that I wasn't crazy and that they just didn't understand what was going on. Eventually, I caved to their demands. I grabbed each of them by the hand and held them tight. I said, "I will do this for you if you can promise me one thing. Promise me that you'll be there when I need you." They agreed.

Some nurses came into the treatment room and informed me they would be taking me to the ward. As we made our way out of the emergency department and down a long hallway towards the elevators, I was surrounded by six individuals. Two were nurses; one was a friend of my sister. She had a concerned look on her face, but I just assumed that she was nervous to be escorting such a powerful being. Who wouldn't be? Two were security guards. I can remember thinking to myself, "how could these two people be in charge of security. If I wanted to, I could kill them with one hand behind my back." The other two were Hannah and Melissa. We made our way to the elevator and descended one floor to the lower level of the hospital. Another long hallway was waiting for us. While walking down the hall, I could see four signs – 1A, 1B, 1C, 1D. These signs were new, but over the next five years, I would become all too familiar with them.

As we approached 1B, we slowed down to a stop and turned left towards a set of double doors. I gave Melissa and Hannah a hug as the nurse swiped her keycard. The light flashed from red to green and one of the doors swung open. I took a deep breath and stepped into a psychiatric ward for the first time. Oddly enough, as I entered, I could feel my irritability decrease. I was still upset that my family had betrayed me, but I knew I was here for a reason and there was much to explore.

A nurse came out from behind the desk and greeted me. One of the first things she asked me was if I had a cell phone. I surrendered it without hesitation as she could see it sticking out of my bathing suit pocket. How was I going to communicate with my team to make sure our plans were still in motion? How was I going to post to Twitter to continue the spread of love across the world? It was okay. I knew they would come to see me. I was their leader, and my troops would come to receive their orders. I was sure of it. After my phone was placed behind the counter, we began a tour of the unit. She showed me where the common area was located. It was a decent size room with tall glass windows on one side. There was a couch with two matching chairs and a wooden kitchen table. One similar to what you would see in your grandmother's kitchen. There was a flat-screen TV shielded by glass and a small kitchenette with a fridge. She informed me that each night they deliver a late-night snack. I looked forward to this as I hadn't eaten since this morning, and my meal consisted of only a couple of grapes with wine. In that moment, I realized just how hungry I was. My stomach growled.

I didn't have a change of clothes, so I asked the nurse if there was something I could change in to. She showed me to the stockpile and handed me a blue robe with a pair of blue cotton slippers. We then made our way to the showers. There was a stand-up shower room and another room with a tub. I noticed old band-aides in the tub and felt disgusted. It was not a tub fit for a god, such as myself. I would choose the shower. I entered the room and the nurse closed the door behind me. As I took off my clothing, I admired my body. I slowly lifted each arm and flexed to test out my strength. I knew that I had many new powers afforded but was extremely pleased to realize that superhuman strength had been added to the list. There was a stack of small towels in the corner. I grabbed three and placed them on a plastic chair just outside of the shower area. I entered the shower and turned on the water. As the stream hit my face, I closed my eyes and thought back to this morning before the police showed up at the beach. I thought of Hannah and how badly I needed her with me. It was the first time in days I felt like I couldn't handle a situation on my own. I wished we had the chance to finish our wine; I wished we finished feeding each other the bowl of grapes. I wanted to finish my work with her and help her ascend into her true goddess form. I felt myself slide into a form of standing meditation and relived that morning with her. We took turns dropping grapes into each other's mouths and took small sips of wine. The sun wasn't just shining on us – it was shining for us. We were the center of the universe.

My eyes opened. Back to work. I had to keep testing my new body. I cranked the water to cold as far as the tap would allow. It hit my body like shards of ice. I could handle it. I grunted loud enough to relieve the pain but soft enough as to not be disturbed. Once I got my breath under control, I cranked the tap in the opposite direction. Scalding hot water smashed against my body. I jumped out of the stream. I felt as if I had been burned by fire. "Come on, Garrett. You got this." I thought to myself.

I held my hand in the water for a minute, then slowly entered once again. I could feel my skin turning red, but I had to prove to myself that I could take the pain. I looked up to the ceiling, closed my eyes, straightened my arms out behind my back and opened my mouth as if to scream. I didn't make a sound, but inside I was howling. I flipped the temperature back to cold to ease the pain, then turned off the water. Enough for one night.

I stepped out of the shower and grabbed the first towel. I put my foot up on the chair and slowly moved the towel over my legs. I was admiring my calf and wondering to myself just how fast I could run now. Was I the fastest person on Earth? There may be others out there who have ascended, but no one has reached the level I have. It would be a fun race between us. Maybe someday we'll find each other and have some fun. I continued with my feet and gently dried between each of my toes. My precision was that of a surgeon. I left no drops behind. I stood up and grabbed a fresh towel for my head. I placed it gently over my face and let my arms hang down by my side, letting the towel do the work – absorbing what it could. I was truly enjoying the process after such a hard day's work.

After I was all dried off, I grabbed the patient robe and put it on with pride. It felt fitting I would be given a robe similar to what the Romans wore; it was meant to be. Perhaps I was meant to be here. Maybe this was a test. I put some thought into the possibility I needed to be here, but I couldn't get past the thought that my team needed me. I decided that it was not meant to be. My family had put me here and that was the end of it. I needed to do everything and anything I could to get back to the outside. I would contact the military tomorrow. Surely, they would understand. They would help me.

I exited the bathroom, threw my towels in the laundry bin and made my way to my bedroom. As I entered the room, my eyes shot to the ceiling. In the center of the ceiling, there was an electronic device with a blinking red light. I knew at that moment that my room was being monitored. They were tracking every move I made. Was this the hospital monitoring me? Was it the military? Or was it a higher level of intelligence? It didn't matter. I knew that someone was watching me, and I had to prove to them they couldn't break me. I got down on the floor and did pushups. I wanted to intimidate them. I did thirty pushups rapidly. I jumped back up to my feet and did squats. I could sense that their analysts didn't know how to handle me. They couldn't believe the power I was putting on display. I was satisfied at fifty. I stretched for about ten minutes, then left my room and headed to the common area. I needed fuel for the day ahead.

On my way to the common area, I passed by a room with a nurse sitting outside of it. She was monitoring the patient. Who was in this room? Was it a fellow infinite? Why were they monitoring them with a nurse when they clearly have the technology to install a ceiling monitor in their room? Maybe this patient was only beginning to ascend to a higher dimensional being and they hadn't reached the top yet like me. Maybe they're worth monitoring so intensely. Perhaps the resources were being spent on me and they didn't have the time to install a device in their room. I said to the nurse, "Hi, how are you? My name is Garrett Campbell. Can I get you anything?"

"No thank you, I'm fine," she whispered. I was surprised that she didn't want me to help her. Here I was, a god standing in front of her offering my assistance and she didn't want it. It didn't really bother me, but I was confused. My only goal was to make sure she knew she didn't have to fear me and I guess I made that clear.

I continued to the common area, entered, and went directly for the fridge. I grabbed a 2L of 2% milk, upset they didn't have homogenized. I grabbed three apples and two oranges. There were already sandwiches on the table. I gathered two Styrofoam cups and brought them to the table and also acquired one tuna sandwich. I filled up the two cups with milk and placed them to my right side by side. I placed the sandwich on my left, followed by the apples, then the oranges. All of my food was positioned in a straight line. I optimized the order so my body would feed off of the fuel efficiently. I started with the sandwich and made my way down the line. I held the sandwich to my mouth and spun it in circles as I bit into to. I would take a bite the moment I swallowed the previous one. There was no time to mess around. This was not for enjoyment. I just had to fuel up. If someone was watching me during my meal, I would have looked like a robot eating food for the first time. All of my movements were ridged and quick. No time was wasted between bites. I can recall taking solace in the fact that everyone in the unit knew not to disturb me while I was eating. They knew I wanted to be alone. After ripping through the oranges, peeling them with my teeth, I chugged the two glasses of milk and let out a loud burp. I was fueled up for the day ahead.

I made my way back to my room, slowly folded the sheets back and slid into my bed. I spent the night staring at the ceiling and periodically checking out the ceiling monitoring device. I didn't want to look at it for too long because I knew it had motion-sensing capabilities, and I didn't want them to catch on that I knew they were watching me. I had to play dumb.

The next morning started with a nurse poking her head into my room and saying, "Breakfast is here." I instantly jumped up out of bed. I took off my robe and chose my dirty bathing suit and wrinkly shirt from the day before. I still wore the blue slippers. Before leaving the room, I made my bed similarly to the way I made it at basic training. Since I was being watched, I wanted to prove that I still had the knowledge from basic. This was a form of basic training. After finishing the bed with perfect hospital corners, I exited my bedroom. I got in line for food and waited for my name to be called. "Garrett!" yelled the nurse. I reached out to receive my meal. I took it into the common room and sat down amongst the crowd. It was a packed room.

As I lifted the top, I observed one hard-boiled egg, a piece of toast with a packet of jam, a small bowl of oatmeal, and a cup of tea. Similar to the night before, this was just fuel. I didn't care what was on the plate. I just knew that I needed to consume it. After robotically eating my meal, I looked around the room. I was scanning to see who was here and if there were any other higher dimensional beings. I couldn't find any. I felt alone. I knew I had to tread carefully or get myself out of this place. After handing in my food tray, I looped all the way around the unit and to the other side of the nursing station. "Excuse me. I need to speak with the Canadian Forces," I said firmly and loud enough so that the nurses could hear me. "Garrett, Dr. Baker is going to see you later this morning and you can discuss anything you'd like with him, ok?" One nurse responded. I replied, "I don't think you understand what I'm telling you! I am an officer in the Canadian Armed Forces and I demand to speak with a representative!" "You're going to have to calm down, Garrett, or we'll have to put you in solitary," she said as she pointed over my shoulder. I turned and looked into a small square room with one small window covered in curtains and only a mattress on the floor. I turned back to her, "THIS IS BULLSHIT!"

I stormed off back to my room. I sat on the bed and put my head in my hands – rocking back and forth. Where is everybody? Why wasn't anyone coming to rescue me? I thought back to when I agreed to come into the unit; I thought of when I told Hannah and Melissa I would do this for them if they were here when I needed them. I needed them at that moment. I remembered that I was being watched and tried to drop all emotion. I couldn't show weakness. I needed to display strength. I could hear a nurse walking in the hallway towards my room, so I jumped to the floor and did pushups. She poked her head in the room and asked, "Are you ok, Garrett?"

"Yep!" I yelled, out of breath. She left me alone and I thought to myself, "That was a close one."

I got myself up and spent the next couple hours walking circles around the unit, grabbing snacks from the fridge and interacting with different patients. I thought that if I socialized, it would look good on me and speed up the process towards releasing me. I had to blend in. Eventually, I heard one of the nurses calling my name. I quickly ran to her with excitement. Maybe someone came to visit me. "Dr. Baker will see you now," she explained. My mood changed instantly. It was game time. I had to convince him that everything was a misunderstanding and that I didn't belong here.

When I entered the room, I was surprised to see that my sister, Melissa, was there. There was also a nurse sitting in the corner with a note pad and Dr. Baker. This was my first time meeting him, but we would become very familiar with each other over the next five years. "Hello, Mr. Campbell, take a seat." His first words. My first impression of him was that he was a very smart man. He was finely dressed with a designer suit and wore a bowtie. I was excited by my first impression. A man like this could see the truth. He would conclude that I am not crazy and that I should be allowed to be let go.

He asked me what had been going on lately. I gave him the same story I had been giving everyone else. I kept this on a human level and didn't divulge any of my newly found abilities. I just told him about the network marketing company and how my friends and I were trying to grow it using the power of love. I explained to him that love is the most powerful force on Earth. We went back and forth having a civil discussion and eventually, he made a request. He asked me if I would consider taking olanzapine to help calm me down. I knew from my studies in pharmacy that olanzapine was an antipsychotic and was often used to treat mania in bipolar patients. I was furious. I thought everything was going so well. My sister tried to chime in that they were only trying to help me, but I could barely register the words she was saying. I felt my heart rate increase and my thoughts raced. They were trying to pin bipolar on me because they didn't understand what was going on. They didn't know that I had an open line of communication with God. They didn't understand that I was no longer a normal human. I had ascended to a higher dimensional being. How could they understand? They couldn't understand something so profound. They explained that I was experiencing mania and that I needed medication to bring me back down. They assured me I was showing the classic signs of mania. They told me I was having grandiose thoughts. I was informed that my lack of requirement for sleep was also a symptom.

My head was spinning. Again, I felt like the walls were closing in on me. I felt anxious. I could barely breathe. I stood up and shouted, "FUCK THIS. MELISSA, YOU DECIDE." I opened the door, stormed out and slammed it as hard as I could behind me. I marched to my room. Within two minutes, the nurse in the corner during the meeting was standing in front of me. She reached out her arms to hand me a tablet of olanzapine and a small cup of water. "Did my sister really tell you to give this to me?" I could barely get the sentence out of my mouth. I was fighting against my tears.

"You just have to trust us, Garrett."

I said, "Whatever," grabbed the tablet and put it in my mouth. I was crushed. I grabbed the water, poured it in my mouth, tilted my head back and swallowed. They had won.

The nurse said thank you, took back the cup and exited my room. I wouldn't see her again until five years later during my fifth episode – the episode where I truly lost control.

After about ten minutes, Elijah and Melissa entered my room. They had a pair of clippers with them and offered to shave my head. They knew I hated when my hair grew for more than a week at a time. Ever since joining the military, I liked to keep it buzzed. "Hey, Garrett, would you like us to shave your head," they asked. I looked up at the monitoring device on the ceiling.

"Sure," I replied. They grabbed a chair, plugged in the clippers and I sat down. They tried to make conversation, but I was too upset to converse with them. Halfway through the shave, I could feel my energy level depleting. I tried to lift my head toward my sister, but I could barely summon the strength. I felt my body keel over. I fought against it and sat upright. I could hear my family snicker at each other. They were happy to see me struggle. Elijah kept shaving. My eyelids grew heavier. Where was my strength? I tried hard to focus. I couldn't. I closed my eyes and let my body collapse. They both grabbed onto me to hold me up and stop me from falling to the floor.

They said, "Let's get you in bed, Garrett." I couldn't fight against it anymore. I let them guide me towards the bed. I tried to speak, but my words were slurred. Elijah laughed at my attempt. They placed me in bed successfully. I could barely summon the strength to move the blankets over myself. Just as my eyes were closing for the final time, I took one last pathetic look at my sister. She was smiling from ear to ear. I thought to myself, "what an evil bitch." I passed out. The olanzapine beat me.

Many hours later, I woke up. I felt hungover. I could barely open my eyes. My mouth was dry. My tongue was like sandpaper. I sat myself up on the edge of the bed. I looked at my hands. I felt weak. I looked up at the motion senor on the ceiling; it was still blinking. "Bastards," I thought to myself. My vision was foggy, and my thoughts felt slow. No, it couldn't be. I wasn't receiving any messages. My line of communication with God was destroyed. I thought of the smile on my sister's face. She knew all along what she was doing. How could she take this away from me? I dropped down to the floor and sat in a meditative position. I closed my eyes. I knew I could get it back. I focused with everything I had left… nothing. Did God leave me? Would he ever come back to me? Surely, he knew that I had no choice; I had to take the medication. I was filled with regret. Why did I succumb to the wishes of mere mortals? I jumped to my feet and ran to the bathroom. I splashed cold water on my face to wake myself up. After three bursts of water, I stared into my eyes. I could see deep down I still had the power. The olanzapine must be interfering with it.

After staring into my eyes for a few minutes trying to figure things out, I noticed that I was still wearing the same dirty bathing suit and wrinkly shirt from the day before when my family turned their backs on me. I looked down at my feet; I was barefoot. Surely my sister left me some fresh clothes. I ran back across the hallway into my bedroom. I looked around. Nothing.

I could feel my irritability return. I marched to the nursing station and asked, "Did anyone leave anything here for me?"

"Let me check for you, Garrett," one of the nurses replied. She came back after a few moments empty-handed and said, "We only have your cellphone back there." My anger grew. I ran down the hallway and grabbed one of the patient phones. I called my brother, Logan. He answered, "Hello?"

"Hi, Logan, it's Garrett. You realize I'm in the hospital, right? That I'm in the FUCKING PSYCH WARD!"

"Uh, hi, Garrett. Yes, I do." He was nervous. "Don't you think it would be a good idea to bring a family member some FUCKING CLOTHING if they're in the hospital wearing FUCKING RAGS?"

"Yea... I guess," he stuttered.

"Then why don't you FUCKING DO SOMETHING?"

"OK!" He finally showed some emotion. I slammed the phone down.

I turned and ran back to the nursing station. "My brother is going to show up here with a bag of clothing for me. I don't want to see him. Just take the clothes and tell him he's not welcome here."

A nurse replied, "That's perfectly fine, Garrett. You have the right to choose who can visit you." "

Is that right? Then I don't want ANY VISITORS!" I screamed. I could feel my power returning. I tried to breathe and calm down. I didn't want them to take it away from me again.

I moved away from the nursing station and walked around the unit on the circular track. I didn't know what to do. I loved my family so much and wanted to see them, but I couldn't get past the fact they were trying to destroy me. Then it dawned on me. I didn't have to rid all of them from my life; I just had to choose wisely. On my way around the track I stopped at the nursing station again and asked to borrow some paper and a pen. They gave it to me. I ran to my room and jumped onto my bed. I drew a grid on the piece of paper and started to write down all the names of my family members. I wrote down the names of everyone who was at the bungalow on the day they called the police in one column and all other family members in the other. Now I knew who I could trust and who was against me.

After my work was complete, I determined that I could trust my godparents, Mary and Donald, as well as my uncle Lucas and my aunt

Ava. I ran to the phone and called Mary and Donald first. I told them I was in the hospital but that I was ok. I told them I needed to see them as soon and possible. I called Lucas and gave him the same information. I couldn't get myself to call Ava. I didn't want her to see me like this. I knew she loved me too much. It wasn't the right time. I ran back to the nursing station and edited my visitor list. Everything would work out after all. I knew they would save me. My power increased, but I still wasn't receiving any messages telepathically. I was concerned because I thought that once I made progress toward my escape, the line of communication would reopen. Perhaps I hadn't done enough. I had to keep working.

I hurried over to the private visitation room and moved furniture. I had to make sure that everything was set up perfectly; this would be the most important meeting of my life. If I could just show Mary, Donald, and Lucas that everyone else was trying to stop me from achieving my goals, surely, they would talk to the nursing staff and I would be released. I moved the table into the center of the room, place four chairs on the far side facing me and place one for myself on the opposite side. I ran over to the bookshelf and tidied it up as much as possible. While I was rearranging the books, I came across some interesting titles. I realized quickly that they were important and that they were placed there specifically for me. I wished I had more time to absorb their knowledge, but I had to prepare for my meeting. I would return to them after. I considered the chairs and adjusted them to ensure that they were in perfect alignment. I looked at the legs of the table and made sure that each leg hit the floor on the intersection of floor tiles. I stood up tall, took a few steps back and observed. It was set.

I left the room and closed the door gently. I took a few steps to my right and swung around. I spread my legs shoulder width, folded my arms, puffed out my chest and remained in my power pose. I was facing the doors to the unit. I stood there for about thirty minutes, waiting for my guests to arrive. I was checking the clock to my left periodically. Just as the second hand of the clock hit twelve, I could see my uncle through the long rectangular pane of glass. I was so content at that moment. I felt enlightened. "Can you please buzz in my guests?" I said to the nurses. One reached under the counter, pulled the lever, and the red light flashed to green; in came my uncle. He came with his wife, Amelia. I was concerned for a moment because I was expecting my godparents as well. Where were they? Surely, they wouldn't leave me here alone. I knew they loved me and would come to see me. Did somebody get to them? Did somebody stop them?

"Hi, guys! Welcome!" I reached out and gave my uncle and Amelia a hug. I could feel my power grow. Soon enough, I would be free. "Come right this way!" I lead them into the visitation room I had prepared perfectly. I knew they must have been impressed. "Have a seat!" I sat them down on the far side of the table and walked around to the single chair. I sat down, leaned forward and put my arms on the table. I started the conversation, "So guys, I bet you have a lot of questions for me, huh?" My smile was enormous. I was confident beyond comparison.

"What's going on, Garrett?" asked my uncle. "Well, you see. I started a new business. It's a lot to explain, but I'll try and share what I can. I started working with Arbonne about a month ago and have been doing insanely well with it. I broke some records for sales in the first month. I built a strong team and we discovered something pretty special. How many people do you know that use shampoo? Everyone, right? Well, listen to this. We're using the power of love to spread our message. It's called Elite 8 Lifestyle. When someone joins our team, they start off with $1500. Now think about it. How many people do you know that you love and use shampoo? If you can find 666 people that love you and you love them back that also use shampoo… That's $1,000,000 in sales. Now here's why we're so good. We're starting with a team of eight people. Each of us only has to find 83 people. What do you think about that?"

The room was silent. Lucas and Amelia looked at each other, then slowly turned their heads and looked back at me. Lucas asked another question, "Garrett, why do you think you're here?"

"Isn't it obvious? I found a way to make millions of dollars and the family is jealous! They're trying to stop me from achieving my goals in life. They just don't understand how big this is! Once the money starts flowing – and it will flow – we're going to start donating it to charity! I'm going to donate $1,000,000 to the Soldier On program and put a leg back on every soldier who lost one in Iraq and Afghanistan!" I explained. My emotion was building. I was fighting off tears. My passion was sincere.

"Why do you care so much about the Soldier On Program all of the sudden?" asked Amelia. "Don't you get it? Everything we have is because of the soldiers that deploy and fight for us. Without them, we'd have nothing. They give their lives for us. We can at least support them with money and love!" I could tell by the way they were looking at me they were concerned. I burst out into tears. I could no longer speak. The passion and emotion were too profound. I cried like a screaming child.

"Everything is going to be okay, Garrett. We think you really need to listen to the advice of your doctor and nurses. We can tell that you're extremely stressed and on edge." I was done. I had nothing left to say. Someone got to them before they came to see me. It was the only plausible explanation.

A nurse poked her head in the room, "Visiting hours are ending in five minutes." I stood up, wiped my eyes and opened the door. Lucas and Amelia stood up behind me. We went out into the hallway and slowly made our way to the exit door. I turned around. They hugged me and told me they loved me. I didn't believe them. I told them I loved them. I didn't mean it. The light flashed green and they exited the unit. I was alone again. I thought to myself, where was Hannah? Why didn't she come see me today? She said she would be here when I needed her. Did something happen to her? I needed to know, but I was trapped and seemingly powerless.

I eventually sauntered back to my room. Much to my surprise, there was a bag of clothing on my bed. My brother had dropped it off while I was speaking with Lucas and Amelia. I later found out from the nursing staff that Logan really wanted to see me but wasn't permitted onto the unit because he wasn't on my list of approved guests. I felt bad for when I heard that he was turned away, but I knew I couldn't let my human emotions hinder my work.

I looked through the bag. I felt a sense of disappointment as many of the shirts and shorts were brightly colored. I thought back to studying bipolar disorder in school and remembered that one of the telltale signs is that individuals would wear bright clothing and extravagant makeup. I couldn't wear half of these. I eventually found a grey pair of socks, grey shorts, and a black Adidas shirt. "Perfect," I thought to myself. I changed my clothes, made my way to the common area and had a snack. This time we were given bagels. I did some laps of the track around the nursing station to blow off some steam, and as I passed by the front end, a nurse informed me that my medication was ready. I felt defeated. I came to the conclusion at that moment that the only way I was ever getting out of there was to cooperate. I took the medication without causing a scene. I did a few more laps then headed to bed. The medication brought on a strong feeling of fatigue.

"Breakfast is ready!" Again, I woke up feeling hungover. My vision was blurred and my mind was foggy. I got up and put on my black shirt.

I didn't pay any attention to the motion sensing device on the ceiling. No thought of it even crossed my mind. I ate breakfast in the common area then headed back to my room with a new idea. It was clear that my family wasn't going to help me get out, so I would try to get help from the military. I still had the paper and pen I had borrowed to make my list of people I could trust. I leaned over on top of the dresser and wrote a list of numbered questions:

1. Why am I being treated in a civilian hospital and not on a military base?

2. Why was I picked up by regional police instead of military police?

3. Why hasn't the military sent a representative to check on me?

4. Can I be transferred to Halifax and treated by a military doctor?

5. Why am I being treated with antipsychotics before trying rest and sleep first?

6. Why am I in a psychiatric ward instead of a regular unit?

7. Why will the medical staff listen to my family but not to me?

8. How long do I need to stay in here to prove that I am ok?

I drew a heart on the bottom of the page and signed my name in elaborate cursive.

I read the questions to myself and thought they would have to answer me. I took the paper to the nursing station and calmly asked one nurse, "Hi, could you please do me a small favor and send a fax for me? The number is 1-902-555-8756." I still to this day don't know why a nurse would agree to send a fax for a manic patient, but much to my surprise, she said, "Sure, not a problem." I frantically ran down the hallway, swung myself around the turn, and darted towards the patient phone. I picked it up and dialed the CFB Halifax Pharmacy. After one ring, someone answered, "Pharmacy. This is Becky speaking." "Hi, Becky, it's Garrett. I need you to do me a favor. I just sent a fax to the pharmacy and I need you to get it and place it on LCdr. Morrison's desk."

"I don't think that's a good idea, Garrett." I could tell she was very hesitant. I had to push her.

"Becky, please. I need you to do this. I'll never ask you for anything again. I just have some questions that need answering."

"Uhh... ok, Garrett. I'll put it on his desk. I think I see it coming through now. How are you feeling?" I could feel my excitement build.

"Thank you so much, Becky! I'm doing great!"

She replied, "Ok, Garrett. Take care of yourself." I hung up. Finally, help was on the way.

Proud of myself, I walked back towards my room. As I passed by the nursing station, they informed me they were going to move me into a different room and that I would have a roommate. I was very anxious about this. I didn't know if they would be someone like me – a victim, or one of them – someone trying to keep me down and suppress my powers.

A nurse led me to my room and helped me gather my belongings. We walked down the hallway, around a turn and skipped three rooms. We entered the fourth room. There was a man lying on the bed closest to the door. The nurse and I placed my belongings on the other bed and she left us alone. I sat on the bed, facing my new roommate. He had his back to me. I sat in silence for about ten minutes until I worked up the courage to say something. "Hey, man. What's your name?"

"Don't trust them," he replied.

"The nurses or the doctor?" I responded. "Listen to me... do not trust any of them. They're going to put a chip in you. They already put one in me."

I was shocked. "Where did they install it?" I asked. My curiosity was peaking.

"They don't tell you where they place it. That way, you'll never be able to remove it." He sat up, turned towards me and continued. "They use nano chips. Eventually, they'll ask you for a blood sample. They don't give a fuck about what's in your blood. They inject the chip into your bloodstream and it finds an undetectable location. Even if you manage to track it down, it will just move. It studies you while it's inside of you. It knows what you're thinking before you do." I was speechless. I instantly knew I could trust him. He was like me, after all. He was a victim. "My name is Roger by the way."

"So, Roger, if you don't mind me asking… How did you find out about all of this?"

He replied with hesitation, "Do you promise you won't hold it against me?"

"Sure, I'm genuinely curious. I trust you. I needed to know."

Then he told me. "It's because I invented them. I was contracted by Google as the head engineer in the nano bot division. I work from home because they just needed my ideas. Google has the technology to read your mind using a frequency emitted from your computer screen. I just sat in front of my screen and fed them technology."

"Wow." I was amazed. "Did you do all of this for free?"

"Of course not, there is $10,000,000 sitting in an offshore account for me right now. I have to hide out here for a while until the dust settles. China is trying to find me. They want my technology."

We talked for hours. Telling each other all about why we were here and what we were capable of. He even corrected my original thought about the motion sensors on the ceiling of our room. He informed me they were actually infrared heat sensors. I believed him, of course. He helped put my mind at ease when he ensured me I was here for my own protection and that I was part of an elaborate plan. I felt a renewed sense of purpose. As we continued our conversation, we could hear footsteps coming towards our room. We nodded at each other and both laid down. We had to make it seem like we weren't talking. We knew we were already breaking the rules by sharing our secrets.

A nurse entered the room and told me that my sister was here and was wondering if I was willing to talk to her. I agreed. I was still upset with her, but I had something I wanted to ask her. I made my way to the visitation room and sat down with Ashely. I immediately asked her, "Where's Hannah? You both told me you'd be here when I needed you. I haven't seen her yet. Where is she?" Melissa explained that Dr. Baker thought it was best I saw no one for a couple of days and took some time to rest. I was furious. I thought back to our magical moment on the beach when I realized my purpose in life – to serve her. How could I do that now, knowing she couldn't keep a promise? I yelled, "TELL HER WE'RE DONE!"

"Garrett, don't say that. This is for the best." She tried to make sense of it. I asked her where she was, and she told me she went to Margaree to spend time with her family while we all figure this out.

"SHE'S NOT MY GIRLFRIEND ANYMORE! TELL HER THAT!" I lost control. She tried to calm me down, but I was too enraged. I kept thinking to myself that Hannah had betrayed me. She lied to get me into the hospital and ruin all my plans. It broke my heart. How could I ever trust her again if she lied to put me into this place? I stormed out of the room and made my way back to Roger. I felt like he was the only person who truly understood what I was going through.

Later that night I took my evening medication and stuck to myself for the most part. I would have the odd conversation with Roger, but I just didn't feel all that into it. I felt like I was in prison and would never escape. Defeat set in. The medication did its job and knocked me out, providing me with another good sleep.

Over the next couple of days, I continued to take my medication as instructed and continued to have conversations with the nurses and Dr. Baker. Each day I would feel my abilities disappear a little more. I continued speak with Roger. We would have conversations each night, but as we progressed in our treatment and the medication did its work on us and we eventually stopped talking about his inventions or my god-like powers. We talked about normal life and how much we couldn't wait to get back to it. It was fascinating how gradual the change was. I was no longer anxious about people watching my every move. I didn't believe that the censors on the ceiling were heat sensing or that they were even sensors at all. Roger stopped talking about his contract with Google or his $10,000,000 offshore bank account. He was more concerned about when his family would deliver his next flat of Pepsi. We never discussed our old thoughts and conversations again. It was out of lack of interest or embarrassment. I knew that we could both remember them, but they just didn't seem real anymore.

Around the twentieth day of treatment, I really started to feel like myself again. The only lingering part of the illness was the optimism. Everything was still amazing to me. I had no hallucinations, no grandiose thoughts, and no desire to help everyone I came across. I just wanted to get back to normal life. At the time it felt like it would happen soon, but this was my first episode; I didn't yet know about the devastating effects of depression that all too often follow a manic episode. I didn't know that I would want to take my own life just months later.

Around day twenty-five, when the nursing staff, doctors, and my family thought I was pretty well back to baseline. Hannah came to visit me. At this time, I had accompanied off unit privileges, so we went outside to talk. It was a hot summer day like we typically get in Cape Breton during the peak of summer. There were no clouds in the sky, and the temperature was at 27 degrees. She looked cute as always, and it warmed my heart to see her. We went out of the back door of the hospital, through the parking lot and found a nice picnic table to sit at. At this time, I felt no sense of embarrassment because I was still hypomanic but controlled on medication. She could tell, though, when I spoke. Just as she tried to start the conversation, I interrupted her and told her that when this was all over, we would get out of here away from my family. I told her they were obviously trying to keep us apart and that we needed to make a big statement so they would understand that they couldn't get between us. I told her I wanted to marry her. I didn't propose to her, but I made it abundantly clear that someday soon, I wanted to take that step. She laughed and told me, "Listen, Garrett, I think we should just focus on your health and getting to back on your feet. We have lots of time to discuss this in the future. Don't you think it's a little quick? I mean, we've only been dating for a couple of months." I was taken back by her response, but I didn't want to spoil the moment. I agreed with her and gave her a hug. Then I told her I loved her.

We talked for the full thirty minutes I had for my pass and slowly made our way back into the hospital hand in hand. She took me right to the nurse's station, gave me a hug and left. As I watched the doors close behind her, I thought to myself that I would do everything I could to marry her. I felt at the time that she was all that mattered. I rushed back to my room and told Roger all about it. I told him I found the girl I wanted to spend the rest of my life with and he was genuinely excited for me. It was the first moment during my hospitalization I truly felt happy.

I stayed in the hospital for another week and was eventually discharged after thirty-two days. I was discharged without a prescription with the understanding that I would be evaluated at CFB Halifax by military staff upon my return. I was given a couple of days to reset at my cottage, then had to pack up and start the drive back to Halifax. It was a four-hour drive, so I had a lot of time to think. I thought to myself, "How did all of this happen?"

It all began for me back in 2014, during a time when I had just graduated from Dalhousie with a degree in pharmacy and was promoted to a commissioned officer in the Canadian Armed Forces. It was a proud point in my life as I had a lot of pride that I took the leap in 2010 to join the military and was now seeing it all pay off. I can recall sitting in the office one day when I received my first paycheck as a Lieutenant. I excitingly opened my banking app on my phone and typed in my password. I would finally see what I had worked so hard for during my time in pharmacy school. I remember how my heart sunk when I saw the deposit into my account – it was for $1836. Knowing what I know now, that was a healthy living wage, but at the time I became instantly stressed. I was never taught about money or finances by anyone growing up, and when I was pushed to go into pharmacy school, I just always assumed that I would be making something around $3000 every two weeks. I never knew how much the government took with income tax. My mother oversaw finances in my household, but she passed away when I was thirteen, so her knowledge wasn't passed down to me. The only advice I ever got from my father was to always have cash on you in case you see something you want. I was stressed because of my poor money management habits and my false expectations of my salary upon graduation, I racked up a $21,000 student loan. I remember calculating the numbers in my head and realizing that it would take a little bit of time to pay off. This kind of crushed my spirits. I tried to look on the bright side in that most of my classmates were dealing with student loans of $70,000 to $100,000 and that my pay would soon increase after I was licensed and was promoted to Captain. I was in a good spot, but I had no idea of the financial hardships I would endure over the next 5 years due to my diagnosis of bipolar. I didn't know that my student line of credit would soon double during my mania.

Just as I was coming to grips with my situation, a coworker and friend asked me how I was doing from over my shoulder. The first thing I said was, "Man. The government really takes a lot of your paycheck, doesn't it?" He agreed and said he had an opportunity he could talk to me about if I wanted to make some extra money on the side. I felt like it would be unwise to decline as he was a very financially savvy guy who had lots going for him in terms of money coming in. I always believed in taking advice from people who knew more about a topic than I did. He most certainly knew more about money. He said he would drop off some products to me to give a try and then he would later explain the business side of it about a week after trying them out. I agreed, and we went back to work to finish our shift.

Later that evening, he came to my apartment and dropped off a bag. It was full of shampoo, face wash, body wash, toothpaste, deodorant, makeup and other self-care products. He brought me items for both guys and girls as I was temporarily living with my girlfriend, Hannah, and her sister. He told me to use them as much as I'd like and that he would get them back whenever it was convenient.

Hannah and I used them for five or six days and I can honestly say they were the best self-care products I ever used, not that I was ever really that into such products. After those days passed, I got a text from my friend, and he asked me if I'd like to go out for a bite and a beer on him to discuss the business side with him and his girlfriend. We arranged a time and we met. He was really excited to talk to me about the business.

He told me all about the company. It was called Arbonne and I could sign up to become a client of his to simply buy products or I could become a salesperson and sell products to my friends, family and whoever else you could think of. I would be paid in commissions and if I signed up as a salesperson, he would help me launch my business and be there for anything I need. At one point in the discussion, he started talking about forming a team to work together and build a network. Once I heard the word team, I became instantly skeptical and asked if this was one of those pyramid schemes. I had a friend that fell victim to one when we were younger and I didn't have any interest in doing the same. We talked about it in-depth and he addressed all my concerns. This company was different and for many reasons and was not a scheme. We talked for quite some time and I eventually told him I needed some time to think about it. At the end of our night, he paid for the bill and mentioned that it was a tax write off because we were out talking about his business. I thought that was very interesting and it really stuck with me. I could get used to having meals at restaurants as a tax write off.

A few days later, he texted me and asked if I had any time to think about it and I replied that I still was sure; I had some reservations. He asked me if I'd be willing to attend a presentation and the Mercedes Benz dealership near my apartment. A National Vice President with the company did presentations there regularly. I agreed as I still had some unanswered questions and was truthfully still interested. I really did want an extra source of income, so I thought I should give it a chance.

We went to the presentation on a Thursday night, and I was instantly inspired by the presenter's story. She was able to retire from her career as a teacher and, based on her level within the company, was making at least $10,000 dollars a month. I spoke with her for a while after the presentation and decided in my mind during the conversation. I was in.

After we left the presentation, we headed back to my friend's apartment to set up my account. He helped me select all the items I would need for myself and some that I would use to lend out to people for testing. The order came to a price of $1500. I had a strange feeling come over me when we submitted the order. On the one hand, I was excited to get started and was still on a high from the inspiring story I had just heard at the dealership. On the other hand, I felt some pressure and I felt stressed that I had just added to my debt. I needed to make this work. I was confident in the business model and was told I'd have the help of my friend and from the National Vice President I had just met. Knowing that made me feel a bit more secure, so I parked my anxiety and let my confidence grow.

About seven to ten days later, I picked up my order. It came in two large boxes. I brought them back to my apartment, where Hannah and I ripped them open. There were so many products. I could see the enjoyment in Hannah's facial expressions as she looked at each item. She loved self-care products and was seemingly in heaven. It made me happy to see her excitement. I texted my friend and let him know that it arrived. "Are you ready to get to work?" he asked. I replied, "Let's do it."

He instructed me to list some people I could contact and present the information to. The first person I thought of was my best friend, Noah MacLean. He was also in the military but was living away in Quebec. We haven't been speaking as much as I would have liked, but I saw this as an opportunity to reconnect on a consistent basis and work together towards a goal. I knew that he would want to sign up just because we would be doing it together. I wrote down some other names, but I was laser-focused on getting in contact with Noah. I was feeling motivated but also a bit overtired. I hadn't been sleeping well since I placed my order and I didn't think of it as a concern. I assumed that I was stressed over the financial commitment I made in joining the company. Work at the base was also weighing on my mind lately as they put me in a very stressful situation, forcing me to temporarily work with someone I had a history with and was hoping to never see again. I found it hard to focus outside of work. These two stressors were making me feel off. I had a bit of anxiety but felt extremely motivated at the same time. I was looking at my goals as if they were more important than usual. I felt like I had a strong purpose in life all of the sudden. My anxiety mixed with motivation was a new feeling for me, but I didn't know I was moving towards mania for the first time. I wasn't yet at the stage of hypomania, but thinking back to how I was acting and the thoughts in my mind – it was definitely the beginning.

I made my way over to my friend and now business partner's house and we called Noah. I was elated to see we answered instantly. He was actually in Sydney at the time and he was at a pool party. I could tell he was happy to hear from me and that he was enjoying himself. "Hey, G bi! Let's switch to FaceTime!" he said. We switched over and I got right to it.

"Noah, man. I got something exciting to talk to you about. I just joined a business with my friend the other day and I'm pumped about it. I really want to work with you."

"That sounds awesome. What is it?" he asked.

"The company is called Arbonne. They sell stuff that everyone uses on a day to day bases like shampoo, body wash, toothpaste – all that day to day self-care stuff. They actually sell fitness stuff like protein and green powders. They pretty much have everything you need to be healthy. We can work together as a team to build our businesses and it's pretty crazy, but when you get to the fourth level, a National Vice President, they actually pay for you to lease a white Mercedes Benz. It's nuts, man."

He laughed and replied, "They give you a Mercedes? I definitely want a Mercedes, G. Look, obviously, I'd be super pumped to work with you and try and build something together. I'm at a pool party right now, so let me just run over to my grandparent's place so we can talk more. I'm just next door, so it'll only take a second. Stay on the line with me."

Noah ran over to his grandparent's place and was laughing, talking about how awesome this sounded. He kept saying things like, "Picture how great it's going to be when he both have Mercedes Benz's!" I was feeding off of his excitement. I could feel a boost in my energy level. He arrived at the house, went inside and sat down. We talked about all of the details about the business. We discussed what was required to sign up and what our plan would be moving forward. We must have chatted for about an hour. The whole time, he just kept saying how happy he was that we could work together on something. He truly was my best friend and it felt good to hear him say these things. At the end of the call, he took out his credit card and placed an order for $1500. His profile was set up and he was part of the team. I had signed my first consultant and was in business with my best friend. I was ecstatic.

We ended the call and Zack and I celebrated my first signing with a cold beer. I told him I felt like I could sign anyone I know. It was more about getting to work with friends than it was about the products. Don't get me wrong, the products were top quality and truly a healthy option compared to others on the market, but the chance to build a business with friends was paramount. I felt so confident in my path. I felt like I found my purpose. My enthusiasm and optimism were growing minute by minute. I told Zack this was only the beginning. We finished our beers and I left to head home.

When I got home to my apartment, I wrote down a list of some names I would contact. I put Noah at the top and instantly put a line through his name. Hannah came out of the bedroom and asked how my day was. I told her all about how awesome our conversation with Noah went that he signed up to build a business with us. She was smiling because she could tell how happy I was. She asked if I was coming to bed soon, and I said I would be there soon. In my mind, I knew I had too much to do, though, and that I would be staying up late. I figured she would fall asleep soon and I would have my space to work uninterrupted.

I stayed up until about 3:00 am that night. Going back and forth from looking at the products to writing down contact names. For some reason, I felt I didn't need sleep. I felt like what I was working on was too important to waste time in bed. Even when I eventually got into bed, I remember just tossing from side to side, waiting for the next day to begin.

When my alarm clock went off, I was already awake and waiting for it. I sprung out of bed and did my normal routine – shave, throw on my military uniform and eat some breakfast. I headed out the door to work with a renewed sense of optimism. I felt like I had a strong goal to work towards and that my future was bright. During my shift that day, I remember having a strong urge to tell everyone what I was up to. I felt like they would want to share in my excitement. I talked about Arbonne with Zack here and there when we had a moment, but I kept it to myself when in conversation with others. I couldn't wait to get off of work and get back to building my business.

During lunch hour, I messaged people on my contact list. I spoke with a good friend, Bruce, and he agreed to meet up soon to talk about it. He said it sounded very interesting and that he was looking forward to it. I told Zack right away, and we decided that he would join in on the meeting as I was yet to do the presentation. Zack also mentioned that the National Vice President had her monthly meeting in a couple of days and that I should really go with him. I didn't need any convincing; I wanted to get more inspiration from her. He also informed me I could bring a guest if I knew anyone that might be interested.

When I left work that day, I instantly contacted my friend and financial advisor, Ben. I told him a bit about the business and invited him to the team meeting. He agreed to come with me. Every time someone agreed to talk about the business, I took it as a guaranteed sign up and new team member. With each conversation, my vision for the future grew and I wanted to work harder. I had grandiose thoughts about what was waiting for me in the coming years. I felt like I would be making $10,000 a month in no time. Even though I didn't have a concrete plan, it was already done in my mind. Sleeping less and less each night, my thought process changed daily, becoming more and more aggressive towards my goal.

Two or three days later, Zack and I went to dinner with Bruce. We talked about the business while we had a couple of drinks and a bite to eat. During our time together, I kept mentioning how crazy it was that I could expense the meal. I thought that that was all he needed to hear to pique his interest. We headed to Zack's apartment afterwards to do a formal presentation. The presentation went well. It was done by Zack and his girlfriend. Afterwards, we asked Bruce about his thoughts on signing up. He seemed nervous and didn't want to commit to anything on the spot. Any concern he had was addressed by myself or Zack. I wasn't willing to take no for an answer. In my mind, I thought this opportunity was the best thing for him and quickly dismissed his need for time or any negativity about joining us. After addressing all his doubts, he mentioned that he didn't feel comfortable putting $1500 on his credit card on the spot. I instantly told him he could use mine and pay me back when he felt comfortable. I felt like I had to do whatever it took to have him join. I knew we'd be making so much money soon this expense wouldn't matter in the long run. We went back and forth, and despite his obvious discomfort with the situation, he begrudgingly agreed to sign up. I felt a wave of power and confidence flow through my body. I was doing it. I was on my way to becoming a National Vice President.

We placed his order, talked a bit about a game plan and then he left to head home. I stayed behind at Zack's for a while and we celebrated another signing. I told him I had a guest for the team meeting and that it was a guarantee that he'd be joining us. He mentioned that while we're at the meeting, we should talk to the host about joining us on a trip to Cape Breton and having a launch party for all our businesses. We would invite as many people as we could and get all our family involved in the party. I remember thinking to myself that I would be able to get twenty people to sign up in one day. It would be easy. I would break every record ever set by the company and be the fastest person to ever reach the top level of management. My vision just kept growing. Even though I only had a team of three people, including myself, I felt like I was a great success. Everyone in my family would be so proud of the work I was doing. Soon I would be able to give my family money and make their lives less stressful. I had thoughts of buying my family homes and cars. For some reason, these thoughts felt normal . I had no experience with Bipolar Disorder, so I didn't realize that signs of hypomania were coming through. I simply took these thoughts as if they were my own and ran with them.

Several days later, it was time for the team meeting. I picked up my friend, Ben, and we made our way out. It was about 20 minutes outside of Halifax. When we arrived at the home, there were cars parked all along the road and the large driveway was full. We got out of the car and made our way up the driveway. Near the house, there was a white Mercedes Benz parked for all to see. I explained to him this was given to her because of her success in the business. I could tell he was impressed, and his interest was spiked. We opened the door and walked in. Instantly we were both shocked at how many people were attending. There were rows and rows of chairs set up and the room was completely full. It was an extension built onto the house and was clearly set up for her business. There were at least 30 guests crammed into the space. There were no seats left over, so we made our way to the back corner and stood to watch what was happening. The NVP was giving the presentation for guests who didn't know about the business yet, and then Zack and his girlfriend got up to do their own presentation afterwards. I was proud of him for getting so involved. After the presentations, the NVP gave out monthly awards to people for meeting sales goals. Everyone would give applause for the recipients and it truly did feel like a caring atmosphere. While I was watching everything happen, I started picturing myself having my own team meetings and giving out awards. I felt like I would be a strong leader and would someday soon be able to fill up my own space. I couldn't help myself. I had to say something. I spoke up and yelled, "Excuse me, everyone!" I introduced myself and my guest and gave an impromptu speech about staying motivated and working harder each day than the last. It was totally uncalled for, and in a usual setting like this, it would more often than not be considered inappropriate to steal the spotlight like that. Not in this crowd. Everyone loved it, and they clapped when I was finished speaking. This only fueled my energy and drive.

She finished giving out her awards and the evening slowly ended. I stayed back afterwards with my Ben, Zack and his girlfriend and we spoke with the NVP. The conversation quickly focused on Ben, and if he was ready and willing to join the team. He was caught up in the hype of the evening and had some good conversations throughout the night with other guests. He mentioned that he couldn't really afford to sign up for the $1500 amount at the time. I told him not to worry about it and that I'd spot him until he could pay me back sometime. I was so confident that we would be making thousands of dollars a month soon, so it would be easy for him to pay me back then. He agreed that he would let me use my credit card for his account, and he got his order placed. I now had a team of four and the support of Zack and the NVP. I felt unstoppable.

It's amazing to think back to my mindset that night and compare it to reality. I thought I was already making large amounts of money and that I would soon be rich. I still had a $21,000 student loan and just put $4500 dollars on my credit card in the matter of days. I was so focused on building a team. If I built a team, the money would come. Although some of the signs of hypomania were pushing through, no one knew to look out for anything, and my intense spending was spread out among different individuals. No one could see the big picture.

On the drive home that night, Ben and I talked about how amazing of an experience it was. We never saw so many happy people directed towards the same goal and seemingly loving every minute of it. He shared with me he met some people that said they needed a financial advisor and that he gave them his contact information. Everything seemed to work out great. He was able to start a new business with me and gain some momentum for his financial advising business. I was happy for him; I was happy for both of us.

When I got home that night, I starting working on my list again. Hannah asked if I was coming to bed, but I told her I had too much work to do. She persisted and eventually got me to agree, but once she fell asleep, I snuck back out of bed and went out to the main living area. I paced back and forth for hours thinking of how I could do things faster. I needed to blow this thing up and I needed to do it now. I was thinking this business was the most important thing in my life and in the lives of my family because it would allow me to change our circumstances forever. I thought of how I would buy my father a new truck and take him to Scotland like he always wanted. I pictured myself giving my sister a check for education funds for the children she was planning on having. I imagined buying Hannah the house of her dreams. I stayed up all night and snuck back into bed just before my alarm clock was set to go off. I was paranoid that Hannah would try to slow me down if she knew I was staying up instead of getting some rest each night. I didn't need rest.

I got up and got ready for work that day, and while in the bathroom, I found myself staring into my own eyes in the mirror. I had a sensation I never felt before. I knew I was tired, but I had an intense feeling of energy. I was so optimistic about everything. Just a week ago, I was stressed about finances and now, even having spent so much money on my credit card, I felt like I was liberated. I remember questioning what was going on with me while I stared at myself. I did my regular routine and headed out the door to work. I had one more shift before I started a two-week vacation.

This time at work, I couldn't help myself but to share what I had been doing. I told some close colleagues that I started a new business with Arbonne and that I was absolutely killing it. I bragged about how many people I signed and about how much money I would be making in no time. They didn't give me the reaction I wanted and some seemed a bit concerned. It didn't matter to me. I was focused on my goal and no one could convince me I couldn't achieve it.

I was extra kind to each patient that approached the pharmacy counter throughout the day. I would spark up conversations with them after counselling them on their medication. I just wanted to be social. I felt like everyone would want to talk because I was radiating such energy and happiness. I was on a high I didn't think I would ever come down from. I would continue to push forward until I reached my goals with my friends.

After work that day I visited the next person on my list, William. I hardly talked about the business in detail at all with him. I simply used my excitement to build his interest. We talked for thirty minutes or so, and then I told him he had to sign up. I said that he didn't even have to worry about placing the order and that Zack and I would do it all for him. He made it clear that he wanted to work with me and was loving my energy, but he didn't have the room on his credit card to place the $1500 order. Once again, I said not to worry about it and that I would put it on my card. We would make money so fast he could pay me back when he started collecting checks or whenever he had the money. He hesitated for a moment. I could sense he wasn't sold so I gave him one more push. "Come on, man, let's do this together. We can kill it. You won't regret it," I said with desperation. "Okay, G, let's do it," he responded. Just when I thought my energy level couldn't get any higher, I felt another burst. I was so proud of myself. I got on the phone with Zack, added another $1500 to my credit card and set up his account. His order was on the way.

On my way home, I got a call from Noah. He was with another friend, Matt. He told me that Matt wanted to join us and that it's something he really needs in his life right now. He wanted to have something that would connect him with friends and have something to build together. I felt like the stars were aligning. I called Noah and got on the phone with Matt. We chatted about how amazing of an opportunity this was for us. He was serious about turning this into a success. He was exactly the type of person we needed on our team – someone with a vision and goals.

That wasn't all of the good news. When I got back on the phone with Noah, he mentioned that his friend John also wanted to have a meeting about it, but he was in Halifax, so Noah couldn't meet with him. I told Noah I would let Zack know and see if he would give John the presentation. I hung up with Noah and called Zack. I felt so busy. I felt like I was running a real business. My vision continued to grow with every conversation. Zack agreed to meet with him, and he did the following day at a coffee shop. Near the end of their meeting, John told Zack that he didn't have the money to put in a sign-up order. Zack called me to let me know the news. I asked to speak with John and told him that if he would pay me back when able, I would put his order on my credit card. He was very thankful and agreed. Zack closed the deal.

In the matter of a couple of days, we built a team of eight people. We had Zack, Ben, Bruce, Noah, William, John, Matt, and myself. I was elated with our progress. What I wasn't focusing on, though, was that I had put $7500 on my credit card to make most of the orders happen. Anyone that knew me and saw what I was doing would know that something was going on and that I wasn't acting right. The problem was that my actions were spread out among so many people that no one had the whole story. Everyone thought they were the only one I was helping out. They all told me they would pay me back but no one could have imagined how everything would play out. No one could have predicted that the business would come to a screeching halt and that no money would be returned.

Zack called me after the deal with John was done and mentioned that we should have a launch party in Cape Breton as soon as possible. He knew that I was on vacation and he said that he would travel down and even get the National Vice President to present at it. It would be a great way to keep the momentum going and really blow it up. We could get everyone from the team down, do the presentation, and have some drinks. It would be a great time. I told him that I'd contact Noah who was already down in Cape Breton, and we would work out a day to schedule it in.

When talking with Noah, he was extremely excited about the idea. He volunteered his parents' house. They owned a beautiful home on the Mira River with plenty of space to have a large amount of people attend. I thought it would be the perfect location. We wanted to do it quick, so we scheduled it to happen in three days' time. Zack agreed that he could make it work, and after speaking with her, the NVP agreed to present. We were all set. Now we just had to get the word out. We made a Facebook event page and invited anyone we could think of. I told the team that everyone should do their best to make it down from Halifax. Everyone agreed that they could make it accept John and William. Through speaking with different members of the team over the next two days, I could tell that everyone was getting really pumped up about it. I fed off their enthusiasm and my energy level just kept going up as the days went on. The night before the party, I really started acting strange.

I played my usual trick on Hannah, where I pretended to go to bed until she fell asleep. Once I knew she was out, I got up and prepared for the next day. I stared at myself in the mirror for a few minutes telling myself this was my moment. If the event went as planned, I would get everything I ever wanted in life. I gathered up some Arbonne products and using them on myself. I washed my face with the facewash, covered my entire body with a revitalizing body spray, shampooed my hair in the sink, and made myself a fizz tab to drink. After I finished with the products, I got out a piece of paper and a pen and placed it on the kitchen table. Just as I set it down, I had what I considered a breakthrough idea. I ran into my office and retrieved my GoPro camera. I brought it back out into the main living area and placed it so the entire room was captured. I pressed record. I knew that what I was doing was so important that I had to get footage of it. I considered the possibility that someone would want to make a movie about my success in the future when word got out about how successful we all became overnight. I thought this footage would be crucial for the director of the movie to see how everything happened. I then turned to my phone and played music on max volume. I put my phone down, raised my arms up to the side and looked up towards the ceiling. I closed my eyes and started singing along with the music. It was a celebration.

As I was singing along, I experienced a sensation that the music was speaking. I felt like the songs were made for me and that they explained my life perfectly. I grabbed my phone again and browsed through the library rapidly. I was looking for songs I thought embodied my life. Whenever I found one, I would play it for just a few moments then move onto the next. I eventually moved over to the camera, leaned down in front of it and spoke to it. I was recording an audio diary of the events that led to that night and explained how monumental these days would be.

I decided at that moment I would be staying up all night to celebrate. I knew I had to drive to Cape Breton in the morning and a four-hour drive on no sleep wouldn't be smart. I called Bruce and pleaded with him to drive my car down to the party for me. I said that I would leave the door to the apartment unlocked and that he could walk right in in the morning to get me up. I told him I have too much to do and that I wouldn't be able to get much sleep. I said that it would be dangerous for me to drive. He was half asleep on the phone, but he agreed that he would do it and hung up.

I stayed up celebrating until 6:00 am and eventually climbed into bed. I was exhausted and hungry. I couldn't fall asleep. Bruce showed up at 7:30 am and like I instructed, walked right into the apartment and knocked on my bedroom door. In all my life, I can't recall a time I was more in need of sleep. Not even during basic training when we were doing sleep deprivation exercises. I had no physical energy, but my mind was still racing. I had to push through it. "G? You in there?" Bruce asked. I told him to open the door. He came in and laughed when he looked at me. "You look dead, man." He told me. I told him I was up working all night and that I'd be fine. It was hard to get myself out of bed, but I climbed out and walked to the shower. I used as many Arbonne products as I could while

I was cleaning myself. I finished, made my way back to the bedroom and got dressed. We were ready to head out.

We climbed into my Ford Escape and hit the road towards Mira. After only minutes on the road, I told him I really wasn't feeling good. He asked me if I had eaten lately. I admitted that I hadn't, so he said we're going to MacDonald's. He told me I needed to eat something; we have a four-hour drive ahead of us. I appreciated that he was looking out for me. I ordered a Big Mac combo and my stomach growled as the smell registered. As we got back on the road, I kept telling Bruce how dead I felt. He kept telling me repeatedly to just take a bite of the burger. I felt so sick, I gagged. He asked if he should pull over so I could throw up, but I told him I was gagging because of how hungry I was. He pleaded one more time for me to take a bite of something and I finally listened. I devoured the burger in a couple of bites and just as I grabbed a French fry, I turned my head to look out the window and saw a Target sign.

"Bruce, you have to take me to Target!" I begged. I had another brilliant idea. He quickly took the exit off the highway and asked me what I needed to get. As I talked about my idea, I felt better all of the sudden. No more gagging. No more hunger. I didn't even feel tired anymore. My energy was back. I explained to him that when I went to the NVP's monthly awards party at her house, she was giving out presents to people and it created a great atmosphere. I thought it would be a good idea to have presents to give out to show everyone who wasn't signed up what it would be like when they joined. I also wanted to show the people who had signed up how much I appreciated them. I told him I would get them all iPad Minis. It would be a great gift to display at the party plus they could use them to go out and sign people in the future when we're all working to grow our businesses. I felt like a genius.

We got out of my car and walked towards the entrance. I was walking with my chest out and confidence high. I felt like a celebrity. I walked in and went straight for the electronics section. I approached the cashier and said I need five iPad Minis. Bruce was sort of laughing and acknowledged this was kind of nuts. To me, he meant this was amazing, and he could barely believe this was our new lifestyle. The worker got the iPads and brought me back to the cash register. They were about $1100 each so after ringing through five of them I reached for my credit card and prepared to put another $6325 on it. I didn't hesitate for a moment; I knew this was the right move. It was just another step towards my millions. After I was done paying for them. I told the cashier I recently started a business and could use a Target credit card because I would be shopping here a lot in the future. I explained that I didn't have time to sign up for it now because I had to get to Cape Breton for a party, but I would take the pamphlet and sign up later. I also offered her to become our Target contact. She looked a bit confused so I took the opportunity to fill her in. I explained to her that some friends and I have recently started a very successful business and we would benefit from having a contact at Target that we could make our purchases through. I asked her if she had a business card, but she told me she didn't. A feeling of disappointment came over me, but I didn't have time to dwell on it. I reassured her I would find her for my next purchase, grabbed the bag and made my way towards the exit. Bruce was right behind me the whole way out and kept saying he can't believe I just bought five iPads. I don't know to this day if he was concerned or believed that I had the means, but at the time I took it as a compliment. I was the man. I was unstoppable.

We hopped back into my Escape and got back on the highway. I told Bruce all about how great our lives would be after this launch party. I asked him if he had ever seen the show Entourage. He did. I explained that his life would be like Turtle's. He would be a good friend of a rich and powerful man that made big deals happen every day. I told him I wouldn't stop until all of our friends and family were carefree and living the life of their dreams. Just as I mentioned friends and family, I realized that I forgot to invite some people to the launch. I quickly took out my phone and started calling them.

The first person I called was a good friend, Sarah. I didn't explain much about the business to her. I simply told her of the location and that if she cared about me, she would be there. She could sense the anxiety in my voice and agreed that she would do whatever it took to make it. I called my sister, Melissa after Sarah. I told her I had something huge going on that I really wanted to share with her and the family. I asked her to do me a favor and call all our aunts and uncles to tell them about my launch party. Even though it was happening later that evening, I knew that Melissa was the best person to make it happen. She wouldn't let me down. I also asked her to make sure my father was there; I wanted him to witness this moment.

We drove for another couple hours while I made my phones calls. As we came closer to the Mira River, I became really focused. I would show everyone an amazing time they would never forget. It would be the day that all their lives changed forever. As we pulled up to the house, I could see lots of cars parked outside. One of them was a white Mercedes Benz. That meant that the NVP actually showed up. I could feel myself becoming more energetic. It was go time.

As we parked the car, I jumped out and grabbed my Target bag. I approached the house and entered through the back door. When I turned the corner into the main living area, I could see that everyone was there. There were people hanging out in the kitchen, some sitting around the dining room table, and even more in the living room. It was my family at the dining room table. I walked up to them, slammed my iPads on the table and said, "Are you ready for this?" I turned away just as they tried to speak and headed right for the Arbonne NVP. I thanked her for coming and told her how much I appreciated her for making all of this possible. I could see she brought a projector and that some furniture was moved out of the way so she could display it on the wall. It was perfect. She said that we would get started in a couple of minutes and informed me there were some people watching online through her laptop from Chicago. This was music to my ears. We would be put on the map after tonight.

As she took her place front and center of the crowd, I felt like I had to say something first. I ran to the center of the room and began speaking. I bragged to the crowd I had an opportunity so great I had been sacrificing sleep to make it all possible. I gave a shout out to all my friends that joined me in my endeavor. As I was speaking, a new idea popped into my head. I realized at that moment this was bigger than Arbonne and that we had an opportunity to change people's lives in a way more important than just financially. I talked about the backgrounds of everyone on my team. We had military members, healthcare professionals, a financial advisor and more. I announced that we would be starting a group that would raise money for charity and that we would be called Elite 8 Lifestyle. I was glowing with optimism. I pointed at the members of my team calling them elite. I ran over to the table and grabbed my bag of iPads. After taking the first one out of the bag, I gave a short speech about Matt saying how proud I was of him for taking the leap and joining the business. I announced that he would getting the passion award and told him to come get his iPad. I spoke about Bruce next, thanking him for driving me all the way down to Cape Breton from Halifax. I announced the Turtle Award and presented him with an iPad. After making up a couple more awards, I presented the rest of the iPads to my team.

Just as I was finishing my speech, the NVP interrupted me. She seemed a bit flustered. She said it was time to get on with the presentation and took over the spot in front of the crowd. As she spoke, I walked around the room high-fiving and hugging my team members telling them, "We did it!"

The presentation lasted about 30 minutes and afterwards a few girls at the party showed interest in the business and spoke with the NVP about it in more detail. I approached my friends from Cape Breton who were there and asked them what they thought. Some remained quiet with folded arms. Others said they thought it was cool but didn't think it was for them. I focused all my attention on one of my best friends, Carter. I sat him down and the table and tried to get him to picture both of us driving around in white Mercedes Benz's. He explained several times he didn't think it was something he'd like to do so I made one last attempt. I told him to let me put his order in on my credit card and do the work. I would find people to sign into his business. I begged him to let me get him a new car. He remained hesitant so I asked him to come outside. We exited the house and approached the NVP's Mercedes. I opened the driver side door and told him to sit in it. He jumped in. I went around to the passenger side and got in. I told him to just think about it over the following days and let me know. He didn't have to sign up now, but deep down I needed him to work with Noah and I; we were all best friends.

As we were talking, I could hear some noise coming from around the house. All of my team were approaching the car. I got out to see what was going on and they told me we needed to get a team picture. I asked Carter if he would take it. We lined up in front of the car and I told the team to follow my lead. I instructed them to raise their hands to their chest, cross their arms, hide their thumbs, and stick out eight fingers. We were making the new symbol for Elite 8 Lifestyle. In the picture we were all smiling ear to ear. We were truly happy and thought we were going to do something big. Everyone on the team believed we were doing something special. Unfortunately, everyone's excitement was blinding them to the fact that I wasn't acting like myself. They just thought I was excited and would eventually calm down. Little did we know, things were just getting started.

Over the next hour, I had a couple of conversations with different people that may be interested and chatted briefly with my family. I was expecting the event to turn into a party that night, but everyone left except for my team. I wasn't fazed, however. It was all I needed to have a productive night. The last person to leave was the NVP. She sat the team down in the kitchen and told us to remember this day. She explained that we were in a great position to help change many people's lives over the next few years. We were inspired by her words. She said she would be in touch soon and headed out the door.

After she left, Noah told me that he thinks he has someone else interested in joining us. His friend, Steve, was going to come out and he wanted to talk to me about it. He also mentioned that he was going to bring some cannabis with him and that we should have a puff to celebrate. As a Canadian Forces member, this isn't an activity I was supposed to partake in, but in my hypomanic state, I agreed.

We moved from the kitchen into the living room and took a seat on the couch. For a moment, I felt tired, but I couldn't let myself get sleepy. I had to talk to Steve later that night. I reached out into the middle of the floor and grabbed the box of Arbonne products. I took out the face moisturizer, squirted some onto my hands and rubbed it on my face and neck. I then reached for the foot cream. My feet were sore since I had been up on them for days and didn't sleep much. I ripped off my socks and rubbed the cream on my feet. I sat back into the couch and thought to myself how proud I was. I was also thinking how happy I was for the team. I felt like this was just the beginning and that it really was going to be a huge deal for all of us.

After sitting around for an hour or so, I heard Noah coming in through the back door with Steve. I looked over and he held up a joint, signaling me to come join then. I put my socks back on, shot up to my feet, and ran over. We went out back and lit the joint. The moment I had a puff, ideas rushed through my mind. We passed the joint around in a circle taking three puffs each per turn until it was gone. I felt like I was on another level in terms of my energy. My heart was racing, and my mind was spiraling. I told Steve to come inside so I could tell him what we were up to. We stopped in the garage and I paced around in a circle while I explained the business to him. After a brief explanation, I broke it down simply. I told him that if we could find 667 people who use shampoo and body wash that loved us and wanted to support us, we would have $1,000,000 in sales. I informed him we already had eight people and he would be the ninth. If he joined us, we'd have to find about 75 people each and we'd be celebrating the $1,000,000 mark. It would only snowball from there. He instantly told me he was in. He ran out of the garage and went to talk to Noah about signing up.

As I entered the house, Zack and his girlfriend were in the kitchen and they told me they were going to call it a night and head to bed. I could hear people in the loft above Noah's garage, so I said goodnight and went to join the other guys. When got up there, everyone was tired and laying down. I couldn't get myself to lay down, so I stood for a while. I kept telling everyone how excited I was and tried to make plans for the next day. They laughed a bit at my excitement but told me I should really get some sleep. I responded by telling them I was too excited to sleep. I continued to talk to them as they slowly fell asleep one by one and finally Ben told me, "G, man. Please go to fucking sleep." I smiled and grabbed a spot on the couch to lay down. I didn't sleep that night, but I decided to keep quiet and let the team get some rest. I just laid down all night thinking about the next steps. I felt like the team needed some time to celebrate and unwind so I thought it might be nice for us to go to my cottage for a night. Just as I thought of the idea, I remembered that Hannah was supposed to be coming down in two days. It was perfect. We could be waiting out there for her and celebrate together.

The next morning when I woke up, I had a text from the NVP letting me know that a Regional Vice President with the company would be doing a presentation at a local venue in Sydney and that we should go meet her. I told Noah and he mentioned it to his team members. Everyone agreed that we would attend. It was at 5:00 pm so we had plenty of time to get ready. I drove home from Noah's at about 11:00 am and jumped in the shower. Again, I used all Arbonne products. I didn't recall eating since the MacDonald's that Bruce forced me to eat the day before on the drive home from Halifax, so I raided my dad's fridge. There wasn't much there, but I got some food into me at last. After I finished eating, I went right back to thinking about the business. Since I thought I was so much of a success, I considered the idea of leasing a white Mercedes Benz. I thought to myself, why wait to be given one from the company when I knew that I would reach that point shortly? I was excited by the thought of it. I couldn't stand keeping it to myself. I grabbed my cellphone and called the NVP. I told her about my idea and asked her what she thought. I wanted to know if she thought I should go get one. She tried to bring me back down to Earth and explained the reasons she thought I should wait for it. She explained that when I make Regional Vice President and I get to walk across the stage in Vegas, it would make the moment more special for me. It would be a better way to celebrate my success. I agreed, and our conversation ended after I told her that we'd see her today at the presentation. When I hung up the phone, I remember being a bit upset that my idea wasn't supported. I thought to myself that I should go buy a black BMW and show up at the presentation with it to show everyone that I'm going to make my own decisions for now on. No one could tell me what to do anymore. The only thing that stopped me from doing it was that there wasn't a BMW dealership in Sydney. I stuck with the Ford Escape, but the idea of a BMW would resurface during my third episode, so I wouldn't be going too long without one.

I spent the rest of the day in the living room staring at my phone while my dad watched television. Noah came to pick me up at 4:30 pm, and we made our way to the venue. The whole drive up, I continuously talked to him about how successful we're going to be and how amazing our situation was. As we pulled into the parking lot, we seen two white Mercedes Benz SUV's parked side by side near the entrance. We got out of the car and walked right over to them. We started taking pictures in front of the cars and posting them on Facebook. In the pictures, we were flashing the Elite 8 Lifestyle sign and smiling as if the cars were already ours.

After our photoshoot, we went inside. We met the other team members inside the lobby and then ventured upstairs to the event. The NVP was already there and she quickly introduced us to the Regional Vice President. I could feel their energy; they were both very excited to see us there. We chatted for a bit and then took our seats to watch the presentation. I can recall midway through the presentation feeling an overwhelming desire to jump up and introduce myself. I wanted to share my story with the room. I was just feeling so inspired that I felt like I had to express it. I'm happy I was able to contain myself. Enough embarrassment was already on its way.

After the presentation, we approached the RVP to tell her how good of a job she did and then we got some pictures with her. She joined in with us on flashing the Elite 8 Lifestyle sign, and then on to social media it went. We then went to discuss a short-term plan with the NVP. I wanted clear direction from her on how many preferred clients and independent consultants each of us should sign. I told her that whatever number she tells us, we'll get it done. She told us to get 5 preferred clients and 2 independent consultants. We had our orders; now it was time to head out. I invited the guys to come out to my cottage in Big Pond, just thirty minutes outside of Sydney. I explained that we deserved some time to celebrate our success. They agreed. I told them I needed to grab some things at my dad's place before we went out. We exited the building, jumped in our cars, and made our way to my dad's.

When we arrived, I hopped out and ran up the stairs. I opened the front door and ran inside. My dad tried to say something when I came inside, but I was too busy. I barely heard him. My friends came in behind me and waited for me in the kitchen while I gathered my things. Just as I finished getting what I needed to head to the cottage and made it back downstairs, I could see my sister's car pulling up outside. Melissa and her husband got out of the car and came inside. Initially, I was happy to see them, but I quickly learned that they were here to try and stop me from achieving my goals.

Melissa first asked me how I was feeling and what I was doing. I told her I was feeling great and was just about to go to our cottage with the guys. I could tell she was there with a purpose. She told me she thought it would be best if everyone left and that I stayed home for the night. Once I heard her say this, I was enraged. I felt threatened. It seemed like she was trying to slow me down and I really didn't have time for that. She continued and told me I wasn't acting like myself lately and that she was getting worried. Some of my friends began to speak to defend me, but I spoke over them. I told my sister I finally found something that I was good at and it was making me happy. I said that I was acting differently because I have never felt this motivated for success before. Her husband chimed in, "Listen, Garrett. I know you're feeling good right now but come on. You know that this isn't how you usually act. Look at your sister. She's scared to death that something is going to happen to you." My sister started crying while he was talking. As she cried, I became more frustrated. I couldn't understand why she was trying so hard to get me to slow down and give up on my dream. She asked me if I even cared that she was upset. I told her I honestly didn't. I would not let her tears get in the way of what I was trying to accomplish. I told them I was going to the cottage and if they wanted to keep an eye on me, they're free to go out as well. Regardless of what they thought or said, I was going. We talked back and forth for another few minutes. She was questioning if I've been eating and sleeping. I lied to end the conversation. Eventually, after they realized I would not budge, they left. Melissa was very upset while she headed out the door. I couldn't get myself to care. I was too focused on myself and my team.

After they left, the rage stayed with me, I felt even more determined in my pursuit. Once again, I could feel my thoughts racing. I turned to my friends and told them it was time to take this thing global. "We're going to go out the bungalow and blowing this up on Twitter. We'll work together by constantly tweeting and use the hashtag #elite8lifestyle. We're not stopping until it's trending all over the world," I explained. They got pretty excited by my idea and agreed it was the right thing to do. We gathered our things, left the house and hopped into the car. We headed for Big Pond.

On the way out we stopped at a gas station so the guys could grab a package of cigarettes. When we pulled into the parking lot, they argued over who would pay for them and what kind they should get. After about a minute of bickering, I jumped in and said I would buy them. They continued to debate what brand they should get, so I told them I would just get them both. I remember feeling proud that I was in a position I could get the guys what they wanted and relished in the fact that the rest of my life would be like this. I would be able to buy anything for anyone regardless of what they wanted. After I purchased the cigarettes, I got back in the car and looked at the guys and said, "Listen, boys. This is how the rest of our lives are going to be. Whatever we want, we get it. We just have to stick together." I handed them their cigarettes and we got back on the road.

When we got on the highway, they lit them up. Once I got my first smell of the smoke, I asked for one. I had never really smoked before. I tried a couple of times in high school when I was drinking like most guys back then, but I could never really stomach them. I found they always made me nauseous. When I put it to my lips and lit it up, it was a totally different sensation than I could recall from the past. I could feel a strong sense of relaxation come over my body with each puff. I truly enjoyed it in the moment. I liked it so much that when I finished it and threw it out the window. I asked for another one. Steve asked if I was sure. "Give me the cigarette," I said with confidence.

During the rest of the drive, I continued to hype up the coming hours, telling the guys we really had to work hard tonight to blow it up. I told them I would get started now. I took out my phone and opened the Twitter app. I created a new account, @elite8lifestyle. I used the photo of the team standing in front of the Mercedes Benz, flashing the Elite 8 Lifestyle sign as the profile picture. I sent out my first tweet, "Something big is happening in Cape Breton #elite8lifestyle." I could feel the excitement pumping through my body.

We arrived at the cottage after dark and pulled down the driveway. Just moments after we pulled in, my father also showed up. I was happy to see him and thought he must want to party with us after the launch party we had. He clearly seen how successful we were becoming and wanted to share in the fun. This is how I perceived it at the time anyway. My sister forced him to come out to keep an eye on me while she tried to figure out the next step to getting me help.

We spent about two hours sending out posts on Twitter. The guys were all using their own accounts but linking each tweet to the Elite 8 Lifestyle account. We kept it going consistently. With four of us tweeting, it didn't take long for Elite8Lifestyle to auto-populate in the Twitter search bar with just a couple of letters entered. That was the first step to start trending. Halfway through our Twitter session, I realized something profound. We already knew that our goal was to find people who loved us enough to support our business, so why not show the world on Twitter this was really about love and not so much about the products. I told the guys to starting tweeting about things they loved. At one point, I even took a picture with my dad and tweeted out how much I loved him. Each time we would follow our tweet with #elite8lifestyle.

Two hours was enough for the first night. Each of us grabbed a beer from the fridge and went out onto the deck. I told the guys how proud I was of them and explained that we were in for a surprise the next morning when our tweets had some time to work their magic. Just as I finished one guy pulled out a joint and lit it up. I couldn't wait to get my hands on it. I remembered the night before that once I took a puff, more ideas flowed. It eventually made its way to me. I held it up in front of my eyes, wondering what about cannabis made me feel so powerful and intelligent. I kept it still for a few moments, moved it to my lips and took a long inhale. I thought to myself, "Here we go." After two more puffs, I could feel it. I felt like I had superior intelligence again. I felt like the smartest man on Earth. I could accomplish anything.

After we finished smoking, we talked about life in general. One thing led to another and I talked to the guys about how I thought I would have a good chance of becoming the Priminister of Canada if I really tried. I justified it by talking about my rough childhood after my mother passed away and getting through a very disturbing time living with an alcoholic as a father who I pretty well had to take care of as a 16-year-old. I bragged that despite these troubling years, I still managed to study hard and get accepted into pharmacy school. Furthermore, I took the leap and signed up to join the Canadian Forces. I travelled to another country to represent Canada on the basketball court and now I was running a business set to explode. I felt like I was on another level when compared to my peers. I truly felt superior. I was enjoying talking about myself and my friends were eating it up and agreeing with me.

My next thought was that we had to document my life. I figured someday, someone would want to write a book and film a movie about what we've done and as the main character, I would need to have everything documented. I figured audio would be the best way to start, and I could always transcribe it later. I told the guys I had to go take care of something and exited the deck. I walked around the cottage property for about 30 minutes, talking into my phone and detailing my past. I started right around the time in my life after my mother passed away. I was 13. I was very detailed in my description. I talked about the morning I was woken by my aunt in my bedroom at the cottage. I remember waking up to her telling me I should go see my mother. I was full of excitement. I hadn't talked to her in days as she didn't have the strength to wake up. I thought she had finally done it. I thought she was back. I came into the bedroom and my brother, sister and father were already on the bed. I took my place at the foot of the bed. Each one of them had their hand on her. I did the same. My mother was not awake. She was taking shallow breaths and there was plenty of time between each. My aunt and uncle were in the room as well, standing at the foot of the bed. The room was silent. My mother took 9 breaths – only 9. This was the first time I saw my dad cry. He looked at each one of us and said, "I loved this woman." We all burst into tears and hugged each other. Our worst fear had come true.

"Garrett! Get back here, man!" Noah was calling for me from the cottage. I pressed stop on the recorder application and put my phone in my pocket. I made my way back onto the deck and Noah asked me if I've been looking at Twitter. I hadn't looked at it, so I took out my phone and opened it up. We had over 100 followers already. Many of the people were from home in Cape Breton. I was excited to see the support. I grabbed two beers from the fridge and gave one to Noah. We cracked them and smashed the cans together for a cheer.

I called Hannah soon after. She was excited to come down the next day to see me. I was ecstatic for her to be a part of what we were doing. I wanted her to see firsthand how big this would be and be around to celebrate with us. Most of all, I just wanted to be with her. I felt so in love. I was the happiest I've ever been. We talked for a little while and she gave me her schedule for the coming day. She said she should be arriving around supper time. After we hung up, the night slowly winded down and I got in bed. I spent most of the night browsing Twitter to track how all our posts were doing. I eventually got about two hours of sleep.

When the next day rolled around, I got right to work. I walked out into the kitchen and looked out the window to get a view of the property and see who was around. I could see my aunt, Mary, laying on a lawn chair tanning. I went to my car and grabbed the foot cream out of the box of Arbonne products. I walked directly down to Mary and told her I wanted to tell her all about my business. When I talked about the products, I asked her if I could test the foot cream on her to show her how amazing it was. I squirted some onto my hands and gave her a foot massage. I did this for about ten minutes, then asked her if she would come watch a short video over at the cottage. She agreed and followed me over. I put on an inspirational introductory video to Arbonne on my phone and handed it to her. "This is what it's all about," I told her. She seemed pretty excited by the video and I asked her to remember that feeling of excitement when I give the family a presentation in the next few days.

I went back outside and saw my uncle, Fredrick, down by our fire pit. I hurried down and told him about what I was working on. When I explained the basic premise of the company to him, he said, "It sounds like you're scamming people." I took the needed time and explained to him how Arbonne differed from many other network marketing companies and why it was legitimate. I felt like I was wasting time talking about minor details, so I jumped right to the main point of the conversation. I told him I would soon have an unlimited source of income coming in, so if he wanted to see his kids more often, just let me know and I would buy plane tickets to fly them home to Sydney. He seemed a bit concerned by what I was saying, but I didn't have time to explain everything to him. I told him to keep my offer in mind and I made my way back to my cottage.

I grabbed my phone and texted my friend, Phillip. I asked him what he was up to and he replied that he was at work. I told him he should come out to my cottage when he got off, but he didn't commit right away. I called him. When he picked up, I talked about how badly I wanted him to come out and be a part of what we were doing. There was a lot of desperation in my voice. He told me he would do what he could to make his way out. That was enough for me. I hung up.

Even though nothing had changed with the business that morning. I felt like I had accomplished so much through the conversations I had. I had to celebrate these victories. I called Hannah. She wasn't on her way yet, but she said that she was packing up and getting ready to start the drive soon. I told her I needed a favor. I was going to send her $750 and I needed her to go to the liquor store and get an order. I needed white wine; only the best would do. I told her to get a couple of bottles of Nova 7 and Avondale Sky Bliss. I needed a quart of rum and a quart of vodka; the brand didn't matter. I told her to get lots of beer; it had to be Keith's. Then I told her to get creative and get a few things she thought we'd like. I also told her to get whatever she wanted for herself. She asked if I was sure I needed so much and I responded, "Just make sure you get everything I asked for." I hung up the phone.

During the rest of the day, my family was doing work around the property. They started by putting up a satellite dish for cable television. I took a picture, posted it on Twitter and captioned it, "Connecting to the world. #elite8lifestyle." Later, they arranged the benches around the fire pit. I made another post, "Outdoor boardroom #elite8lifestyle." They took a break afterwards and hit some golf balls into the lake. I couldn't resist; I had to share it. I posted on Twitter, "Elite 8 Lifestyle driving range #elite8lifestyle."

Right after I made the third post, I looked up to the cottage and I could see that my sister had arrived. I made my way up to talk to her, but before I got a word out, she asked me if I checked the results of my national pharmacy licensing exam. It was September 7th, and they were due to come out. I had this date ingrained in my mind for the longest time, but with all the excitement, I totally forgot about it. I told her I didn't check yet. "Well, do you think it would be a good idea to check if you have a pharmacy license?" She asked with a bit of attitude. I jumped onto the laptop and brought up the list of new licenses issue. I scanned the list for my number. It was nowhere to be found. I check a second time. I checked again. I wasn't on the list.

The results are set up so you can check a list of people who had passed both parts of the exam. There was an in-person practical exam known as the OSCE where you role play different scenarios with an actor and there was also an MCQ exam that was only multiple-choice questions. If you weren't on the list of people who had passed both, you had the option to check the list for each section of the exam. I checked the OSCE list first and found my number. I had passed it. I moved over to the MCQ list but couldn't find my number. I would have to redo it in six months and would not get my pharmacy license this time around. If I was my normal self, this would have ruined me. I would have had immediate anxiety and felt like a failure. This didn't happen, though. I stood up from the table, and my sister asked me how I felt. I told her it was fine, and that pharmacy doesn't even really matter to me that much anymore. I pointed to my graduation ring and told her, "This is just a credibility ring now!"

"Garrett, you just found out that you failed your licensing exam and you don't care. This is not you," she pleaded.

I responded, "Would you rather me curl up into a ball cry about it, Mel?" I walked away from the conversation and went out on the deck with the guys.

Hannah showed up about an hour later and I ran over to the car to greet her. When she got out of the car, I told her instantly that I failed the licensing exam, but we would not let it ruin our night. I asked her if she got the liquor; she got it all. I gave her a hug, thanked her, and brought all of the liquor inside. I set it up on the kitchen table, took a picture, and posted it to Twitter. "Elite 8 Lifestyle bar. #elite8lifestyle." I told the guys to have whatever they wanted.

Just as I was pouring myself a drink, Noah let me know that someone who works at Apple started following our Twitter page. He shoved his phone in my face to show me. It was legitimate. The new follower did work for Apple. I told Noah to find out what he could about the guy. My mind was racing. I could feel everything coming together, but I felt like I needed to do more. I needed more cannabis. I needed the abilities and higher level of thought it gave me the night before. I asked the guys if anyone had some. Steve had a bag, so he rolled up a joint. We went outside to the back of the cottage and lit it up. Once again, the moment I took my first puff, I could feel my mind change. Everything seemed so clear and ideas flowed. My feeling of superiority also increased. I felt like no one could compare to me. I felt like I was a higher-level human. I could problem solve like no one else could. Any idea I thought of could be easily made into reality. I felt like I had special powers.

As we finished the joint, I could see my friend Phillip pulling down the driveway. I rushed over to his car. I was extremely excited to see him. I knew he would come. He got out of the car and I gave him a hug. "Thanks for coming, man!" I said with a smile from ear to ear. "Wait until you see everything we've been doing to the place, man. It's the Elite 8 Lifestyle headquarters. We have everything, even a driving range. I'm so glad you came." I was speaking a mile a minute. Phillip asked me if I was feeling ok. I replied, "Man. I've never felt so good. I feel like I can accomplish anything. I don't know what's going on with me but let me tell you something. Just keep it to yourself. I feel like soon, I'm going to be able to levitate. Don't worry about that, though. That's not for a little while. Let's go inside."

We entered the cottage and I offered him a drink from our collection. He declined because he had to drive home later. I understood, but I was upset because I really wanted him to participate in the celebration with us. Before he had a moment to speak, I told him all about my day. I told him we set up a satellite to connect with the world and a boardroom for meetings. I told him that the company Apple was following us on Twitter and I also mentioned that all of our friends will be insanely rich when we reach our goal. I didn't get the reaction I expected; he just sort of nodded and barely acknowledged what I was saying. I didn't let it phase me. I knew he'd come around.

Just as I finished speaking to him, two of my first cousins came into the cottage. It was Manson and Elijah. I was happy to see them. "Hey, guys. I'm so glad you came over. It's perfect timing. I need to talk to you guys in the back room for a second. I need you to come too, Phillip. I have something important to share with you." Everyone nodded and followed me down the hallway. We entered my bedroom and I took a seat on the bed. I explained the situation to them. "Listen, guys. As you know, I've been working on something really hard over the last few weeks. It's really starting to blow up and I need you guys to do me a favor. It's really important. Soon I'm going to be very rich and most likely famous. I asked for you guys to come back here because I want you to keep me grounded during all of this. It's going to get crazy and I trust the three of you. I need you to keep me grounded and be honest with me if you think I'm letting it all get to my head. I'll look after you guys financially. I just need you to have my back." They were all staring at me. The room was silent for a moment. They turned and looked at each other, then Elijah spoke up, "Garrett – Are you sure you're ok? Maybe you should have a conversation with your sister about all of this." My anxiety began to emerge. "I'm not talking to Melissa! She doesn't understand what I'm trying to do! She's already tried to slow me down once and I'm not giving her another chance!" I shouted.

I got up and stormed out of the room, feeling like I couldn't trust anyone. I was trying to make the lives better for everyone that I cared about, but all they wanted to do was try to stop me. I went to the kitchen and poured myself a drink to calm down.

The only people I felt safe around was my team and Hannah, so I felt lucky when everyone else slowly cleared out of the cottage. Even Phillip left. I was surprised that he left so soon, but I was a bit relieved. My anxiety slowly dissipated with the now smaller group of people. I told the guys we should do a quick Twitter session before we hang out for the night. We sat around in a circle and started tweeting. After about 15 minutes, I made my final tweet for the night. It was a picture of Hannah and captioned, "This girl follows me through life. You should follow her on Twitter. #elite8lifestyle." In my mind, I just did Hannah the favor of making her famous. Endless amounts of people would start following her account. She could leverage her new following as she saw fit.

We finished the night with a couple of drinks. I spent the entire evening thinking to myself about what new abilities I would acquire next. I already knew that levitation was coming, but now I was thinking about mind reading. I felt like I would soon have the ability to do it. I can recall going into the bathroom that night and looking at myself in the mirror again; I stared at myself in the eyes. I was confused as to what was going on with me, but I didn't care to figure it out. All I knew was that I've never felt so alive. I felt powerful. I felt like nothing could stop me from achieving anything I set my mind to. Again, I thought to myself that I was a higher level being; I was an infinite human.

Hannah knocked on the bathroom door asking me what I was doing. I didn't realize that I was in there for over 10 minutes. I opened the door and gave her a hug. She told me she wanted to go to bed and that I should come with her. The last thing I wanted to do was to go to bed. I felt like the longer I stayed up, the more powerful I would become. I didn't understand why that was the case, but I knew it to be true. I knew I had to go with her, though. She had travelled all this way to see me so the least I could do was sleep with her. I knew deep down I would most likely not be able to sleep again, but I could lie with her and rest. I really wanted to go out with the guys and blow up Twitter all night. I wanted to share what we were doing with the entire world and speed up the timeline to our success. I told the guys to enjoy the rest of the night and headed down to the bedroom with Hannah.

When I got into bed, I felt so energetic; it was hard to lay still. I kept hugging Hannah and talking to her about how great of a life we would have. She asked if I've gotten any sleep lately and I bragged about how I didn't need it. She then told me I should really try and get some rest tonight. I felt a little threatened by her persistence so I decided that I would try my hardest to lay still all night so she would think I slept. She didn't know what I was. She was unaware that infinite humans didn't need sleep.

I spent the night lying still in bed with my eyes closed. It was hard not to get up and do more work but I stayed put. While lying there quietly, I felt like I was in a form of meditation. I felt like I could remove myself from my body and travel to other places. At one point, I really concentrated and pushed myself out into the universe. I was talking with different types of beings from all over different galaxies. They were all kind and wanted the best for me. I assumed this was how infinites communicated with each other. It was nice to see so many beings like myself out in the cosmos. I asked them if they would come visit my physical body someday, but they said people on my planet weren't ready for such a visit; it would cause too much despair. Although this made me sad, I understood their concern. I then asked them if they had any advice on communicating with the dead. I was told that once I ascend to a high enough level, I could do it on command. When I received this information, I had a pit of anxiety in my chest. I knew it was what I wanted, but I didn't know if I was ready for it. I wanted to speak with my mother. It had been 12 years since I saw her and I thought about her every day. I knew it would happen for me. I had to prepare myself mentally for it.

I eventually dozed off to sleep for a short period and was woken up by Noah coming into my room early in the morning to let me know that he was heading back into Sydney to sign some preferred clients. I asked him to let me know how it went and he was on his way. I woke Hannah up shortly after and gave her a hug. I felt like I had been away during the night even though I was physically there the entire time. I had missed her. I couldn't believe how cute she was when she woke up. I gave her a kiss and could feel the love between us. I was happy. I had so many thoughts about our future together. I would do anything I could to make her happy.

Just as I was relishing in my happiness, I could feel my brain pulse. I turned around to lay on my back and as I turned, it happened. I could see her. My mother was standing in the doorway to the bedroom. She took one step forward towards me and then stood still. We were staring at each other. I didn't want to scare Hannah, so I spoke to her telepathically. I told her I missed her and asked if she was proud of me. She smiled. I then asked her if she would stay with me. I didn't want her to go. I was sick of living my life without her. Everything was so easy when I had her in my life. She didn't answer me. Instead, she turned around and looked up the hallway. As she stood there, I could hear someone coming down the hallway. My aunt entered the bedroom and my mother was gone. She vanished.

My aunt asked me how I was feeling this morning. I could barely get myself to respond as I was irate that she made my mother leave me.

There were so many questions I wanted to ask her, and I just wanted to spend more time together. I responded to my aunt by yelling at her, "What the fuck gives you the right to storm into my bedroom like this?"

She was taken aback by my aggression. "Garrett, yesterday you were acting different than you normally act. Your family is really concerned about you. You need help," she pleaded. I screamed back at her again and told her to fuck off. I stared at her in the eyes while I shouted it. She turned around, left the bedroom, and stormed down the hallway. I could hear the door close behind her as she left the cottage.

I had a sudden burst of energy during the encounter, so I got out of bed and went out into the kitchen. I wasn't hungry, but I knew I had to feed my physical body, so I opened the door to the fridge and piled anything I could find onto a plate. I stuffed my face with food and just as I finished a couple of bites, I could hear someone coming up the steps outside. I looked out the window and saw my first cousin, Elijah, and my uncle, Fredrick. I knew they were here to try and stop me. Rather than letting them corner me inside, I ran out onto the deck to confront them. "What the fuck do you guys want?" I shouted. Elijah said that they were only here out of concern and that Mary sent them over. I told them to get off my step. Elijah tried again to talk to me rationally, but I wasn't having it. I told them to stop trying to slow me down and hold me back. Fredrick tried another approach. He held his fist in the air and told me to calm down before he does something he'll regret. I loved it. I wanted to fight. I wanted to give both everything I had. I screamed, "Come on, Fredrick! Give it a try! I dare you!" I was flexing at them while I yelled. I was truly hoping for them to come at me.

Elijah grabbed Fredrick and slowly walked backwards with him. He knew that it would not do any good talking. They left me alone. I was done entertaining my family. I was furious after the altercation. I went back inside and approached Hannah in the bedroom. I asked her if she would get up and spend some time with me away from everyone. I needed to have some peace and quiet. She quickly agreed. She got out of bed, got dressed and joined me in the kitchen. I told her I wanted to have a picnic with her. I wanted to go down to the beach for hours and let everything blow over. We grabbed two bottles of wine from our liquor collection, then headed to the fridge. I grabbed the grapes and threw them into a bowl. Last, I grabbed two towels for us to lay on.

As we walked across the compound, it really did feel like I was finally being left alone. There was no one in sight. There was only peace and quiet. We walked down over the bank and onto the beach and walked for about 5 minutes to find a private spot. I set up the blankets, opened the wine, and began to finally relax. You know what happened next.

EPISODE 2

WHEN I ARRIVED BACK IN HALIFAX, I WAS STILL FULL OF enthusiasm towards life. All of the hallucinations were gone. I was showing no signs of psychosis. It was just that lagging enthusiasm that stuck with me. Even after everything I had been through, I still believed a lot of what I thought when I was fully manic. It was like I couldn't shake the positive thoughts. Perhaps I was back down to a hypo-manic state and needed more medication to get completely back to level. After now having five episodes, I know that a month in the hospital is never enough for me; I'm always released too early.

When I got back to Hannah's apartment, I walked in and had a flashback of the night before I left for the launch party. I remembered dancing in front of the camera to document the night. I laughed to myself thinking about it. It still seemed normal. Just as I finished my laughter, my phone rang. I didn't recognize the number. I answered. It was the head of the military pharmacy on the line – a high ranking pharmacy officer. He asked me how I was doing and wanted me to give him a rundown of the situation. I explained to him I had just gotten released from the hospital, and during my stay, I was diagnosed with Bipolar Disorder. He expressed his sympathies towards the situation and informed me that due to my diagnosis, he would have to suspend all training immediately. I was supposed to go to Borden, Ontario for a pharmacy officer training course and then head off to Moncton to complete my six-month residency at the Moncton hospital. I confirmed with him that both were to be cancelled and found out that they were. It was kind of a shock to my system as I could feel my career falling apart. I also had to take this opportunity to inform him I needed to redo the multiple-choice portion of the pharmacy licensing exam. It was not a good call for me. Everything felt so on track just a month ago.

As we ended the call, I really felt like I needed some positivity. I felt like I could only get that from my team. I texted a few of the team members in Halifax, asking if they wanted to meet up and make a game plan for how we would move forward. I waited about ten or fifteen minutes for a response, but no one answered. I tried calling them. Nothing. I was confused. I chose to believe that they were just busy and decided I would grab a shower to rinse off the day. When I walked into the bedroom to get undressed, I saw a bag sitting on the bed. I looked inside and found 5 iPad minis. My head started to spin. I thought to myself, "How did these get here?" Hannah had travelled back to Halifax before me, so she must have brought them with her. But why didn't the guys have them? I gave them to them to use to sign new clients and here they were sitting on my bed.

I grabbed my phone and called Hannah. She picked up right away. I got right to the point and asked her why the iPads were all here in Halifax. She told me that Melissa got them back while I was in the hospital so I could return them. She was really concerned with how much money I spent on them. I was furious. Who did she think she was to interfere with my business like that? I hung up the phone and texted the guys apologizing for Melissa taking the iPads. I told them I still had them and would do my best to get them back to them. No one answered my text. I tried calling a couple of them again. I still could reach no one. I was so confused. Why wouldn't anyone talk to me?

I took off my clothes, went across the hall to the bathroom, and got into the shower. I grabbed the Arbonne body wash and scrubbed my body. I cleaned my hair with the Arbonne shampoo. I squeezed some Arbonne face wash onto my hands and scrubbed my face. I looked at the products. A part of me still believed that they would make me millions. I turned off the water and jumped out of the shower. While I was drying off, I could hear Hannah come into the apartment. I rushed to finish drying off and went back across the hall to the bedroom to get dressed. I came out of the bedroom, approached Hannah, and gave her a hug. I asked her what was going on. I wondered why none of the guys would talk to me? She explained that Melissa had contacted everyone and asked them not to talk about Arbonne anymore. She explained that a symptom of Bipolar Disorder is that you often participate in risky business ideas and that they're pretty sure that's what happened here.

I couldn't believe what I was hearing. My own sister was single-handedly destroying my business after all the work I had put in to build a team. I was devastated. Hannah told me this was for the best, but I could barely acknowledge what she was saying. The fact was that I didn't believe I had Bipolar Disorder. I was in complete denial and my mood was still not completely back to level. I tried calling William a few times. He was one of my best friends; I knew he would answer. He eventually did, but when I asked him about Arbonne, he said he had a change of heart and would drop off the order he received to me. I got Bruce on the phone too. He said the same sort of thing. He asked if I could come pick up his products from him.

Over the next hour, I went to pick up Bruce's products and William's were dropped off to me. I now had $4500 worth of Arbonne products and two fewer team members. No one else would really answer me, so I assumed they were all out too. It was all falling apart. Even though I was crushed, I couldn't shake the feeling of optimism I had in my mind. I still felt like I could somehow turn this all around. It was getting late, so I had a snack, prepared my uniform, and got in bed.

Waking up the next day, I was excited to put my uniform on. I missed wearing it over the past month. I always felt proud of myself when I wore it. I made sure my sleeves were perfectly rolled and put some extra wax on the toes of my boots. I left the apartment, hopped into my Ford Escape, and made the ten-minute drive to the base.

When I walked into the pharmacy, I was happy to see everyone, although I couldn't help but feel a sense of embarrassment. They all knew I was in the hospital for a month and were now looking at me as someone with a mental illness. Even though I still didn't believe I had Bipolar Disorder, I could feel how they were looking at me. It was different. The team lead of the pharmacy asked me to come into his office, and we discussed how I was doing. I was still feeling good, so I told him I was just happy to be back and was looking forward to getting back to work. We discussed failing the MCQ section of the licensing exam, but he said it wasn't my fault given the circumstances. We would just look forward to writing it in November during the rewrite. I appreciated his kindness regarding the situation. He told me that I'd have to head up to the mental health clinic as they're expecting me today to do some follow up from my hospitalization.

I knew exactly where to go since I used to go up sometimes to ask the clerks questions about some of our patients. I made my way up to the fifth floor of the clinic and approached the reception area of the mental health unit. I gave them my service number and they told me I would be seeing Dr. Edwards and to have a seat. The waiting area was very open to the nearby hallway, so I felt uncomfortable as many colleagues walked by and noticed me in the waiting area for mental health. I felt like I was below them and that I was being judged. I was always so used to being the health care provider, and now all of the sudden I was a mental health patient in my workplace.

A nurse eventually came to get me and brought me to the psychiatrist's office. I entered the room and took a seat on the couch. We talked for a while about my stay in the hospital, and he explained that I most likely know as a pharmacist graduate that the best thing for me was to start on a mood-stabilizing medication. He asked how I felt about starting Divalproex. I wasn't happy about it and still at that moment, didn't believe that I had Bipolar Disorder. I had convinced myself that I must have had a mental breakdown due to stress over my exam. I was a military member, however, so I followed his instructions and went along with it. He told me I had the option of getting the prescription filled off base if I didn't want to fill it where I worked. Still feeling optimistic, I said it wasn't a problem and brought the prescription down to the pharmacy. I remember joking with one of the technicians as I brought the paper to the window. If felt so strange to be on the other end of the healthcare system. It was odd to feel like the patient rather than the provider.

After dropping off my prescription, I went back into the pharmacy. As I entered, the team lead told me I had to go speak with Dr. Noseworthy. He told me where to go to see her and I did as I was told. I went back upstairs and touched base with a receptionist. I was in her office within five minutes. I went in and sat down and she spoke, expressing her sympathy for the situation. She was very kind and honestly reminded me a lot of my mother. Their physical appearance was similar as well as their mannerisms. After talking back and forth for a little while, she broke the news to me. She told me that due to my condition and my inability to be deployed, I would have to be medically released from the Canadian Forces. I could barely speak. I acknowledged what she had told me but couldn't really think of what to say. She continued and told me it was a long process and said not to get too down about it. I had a good degree and would be fine for work on the other side. I had planned to spend the full 25 years in the forces and make a career out of it and just like that, it was all over. Even with this news, I still didn't believe I was Bipolar. Everyone else was mistaken.

I eventually left the office and made my way back down to the pharmacy, where I finished out the day. My prescription was ready as I was leaving, so I grabbed it off the shelf and made my way out. When I got home, I explained the situation to Hannah. I was frustrated, but I couldn't shake the feeling that everything would work out for the best. Hannah told me we would get through this together. I believed her. After we were done talking about my day, Hannah shared with me she found a new apartment for her and her classmate. I was happy for her, but I was a bit upset because I now had to find myself a place to live. The original plan was to live with Hannah until I went off on my training, but now, I would be staying in Halifax a little longer term. It would be at least for the foreseeable future.

Over the next week, I found a bachelor apartment across the street from Hannah's new apartment. It was in a building called Fenwick tower. It was kind of a rundown place, but I didn't care; I just wanted to be close to her. It took me a day to get moved in after I signed the paperwork.

It was easily the ugliest place I had ever lived, but I was trying to stay optimistic. I was close to Hannah and I had cheap rent. Hannah started school in September, and I continued to work at the base.

Everything was going fine for the first couple of weeks, but then my mindset changed. It started one day in mid-September when I woke up and had a sense of feeling alone. When I put my uniform on, I didn't feel as confident as usual. My energy level also felt way down. I brushed it off as a bad start to my day and made it through the workday. I didn't feel as social while I was at work. I kind of felt like everyone was looking at me differently and could tell I wasn't myself. Every day got worse and worse until I had my first breakdown.

I was at work one day and was struggling in my day to day conversations. I thought of myself as a failure because I was waiting to get medically released from the organization I loved. I thought of myself as worthless because I was supposed to be a licensed pharmacist and was waiting to rewrite my exam. I felt disgusted by myself. My vision got fuzzy and I developed a headache. I couldn't get myself to break the thought patterns I was experiencing. Everything was negative. As patients kept coming to the counter, I struggled more and more. My heart pounded and I felt like I had to get out of the pharmacy. I turned to one of the other pharmacists and said, "I need help." She asked if I was ok and I told her I wasn't. She told me I should speak with the team lead. I slowly made my way to his office and asked if I could speak with him for a moment. He invited me in.

I sat down on a chair in his office, hunched over. I felt so embarrassed, but I knew I had to explain myself. I told him, "I really think I need to talk to someone." Just as I finished the sentence, I began to cry. It was only for a moment, but I couldn't hold it in. I couldn't get rid of the feeling of defeat. He instantly stood up and said we had to go upstairs to the mental health unit. I wiped my tears away and followed him upstairs. We approached the counter and he explained the situation. He told them I needed to speak with someone as soon as possible. They asked who my doctor was, and I told them it was Dr. Edwards. They told us to head down towards his office and they would call him. We made our way down and stood outside of his door for about ten minutes. He eventually opened the door and invited us in. He asked me what was going on. I explained to him I had an overwhelming feeling of worthlessness and I can't focus on anything good in my life. "I don't know why but I just feel so sad," I said. Tears ran down my face as I explained to him how I felt.

He asked my team lead to step out so we could continue the discussion. We talked in length about the fact that it's common for patients with Bipolar Disorder to flip into depression after having a manic episode and this is likely what is happening. I understood that from studying it in school, but I just felt so overwhelmed and had never truly felt clinical depression before. I was confused and a bit scared at how I felt. He then asked me if there are any stressors in my life I could eliminate so I could focus more on getting better. The only thing I could think of was the upcoming rewrite for the licensing exam in November. He said that I was in no shape to study and that it would probably be best if we pushed that back for the time being. I agreed that I couldn't focus right now and that it would not be a good idea to write it. A part of me felt like more of a failure for agreeing to push it back again, but I also had a sense of relief. After talking for a bit longer he decided to give me a few days off and to refer me to a psychologist so I can more freely talk about what is bothering me. He printed me off a note for my team lead, indicating my duration of time off. I left his office, dropped off the note, and left the building.

I felt relieved to get away from everyone. I just wanted to get back to my apartment and climb into bed. I didn't want to be awake. I made it back to my car and drove home. As I entered my apartment, it really hit me just how rundown it was. I was optimistic about it before, but now I was dreading being in it. Everything negative was sticking out to me. I wanted to call Hannah, but I was embarrassed to tell her what happened. I was embarrassed that I had to leave work. I took off my uniform and climbed into bed. I laid there for hours thinking about how much of a failure I was. I eventually fell asleep.

When I woke back up, it was dark out. It was around 8 o'clock. I hadn't eaten for a while, so I was starving. I still felt drained of energy. I just wanted to go back to sleep so I didn't have to exist in my reality. I was too hungry to fall asleep, but I was too tired to get up and make food. It was a vicious cycle. I eventually forced myself to get up and stumbled to the kitchen. I didn't want to cook, so I grabbed a banana and ate it. I threw the peeling on the counter and climbed back into bed. While I was lying there, everything that I had done and said while I was manic came rushing back into my mind. I suddenly recalled all the money I had spent doing other people's Arbonne orders for them. I remembered giving a speech in front of all my family and friends about Elite 8 Lifestyle. I wondered why I spent so much money on liquor at the cottage. I wondered why I was using Twitter like a maniac talking about everyone I loved. I sat up and unlocked my phone. I logged into my online banking to assess the damage I had done. I saw the thousands of dollars I had spent. It was all for nothing. Everyone said they would pay me back, but now no one would even talk to me. I dug myself into a financial hole and to make matters worse, I was getting released from the military. I wasn't even a pharmacist yet like I should be. I was a complete failure. I felt like my life was over.

I woke up the next day in the same vicious cycle as the previous night; I was too tired to get up and make food but too hungry to go back to sleep and avoid my life. I was still too embarrassed to tell Hannah I wasn't working. It made me feel worse about myself that I needed to hide out in my apartment. The whole day I could only think of negative thoughts. I focused on my finances and the fact that I had increased my debt for no reason. I thought about the fact that all my family and friends now thought I was crazy after being hospitalized with a mental illness and that I was getting kicked out of the military. I really wanted to make a career out of it. I loved travelling to play basketball. I loved how they would push us to exercise and stay fit. I didn't know what I would do. I was so worried about everything. In that moment, I truly didn't want to live anymore. I thought about how I would kill myself if I was to do it. I first imagined slitting my wrist. I walked over to the kitchen and grabbed a knife. I didn't have the intention of doing it in the moment, but I just wanted to imagine what it would be like. I held the knife against my wrist and pictured making the cut. It gave me more anxiety. I knew I couldn't do it this way.

Soon after, I thought of another idea. I remembered hearing a story of a young girl jumping off a balcony at Fenwick just a few years ago. They had protective nets up now to prevent people from jumping, so I grabbed a pair of scissors and walked out onto the balcony of my 31st-floor apartment. I stood there for a while, thinking about what it would be like to cut the net and jump. I pictured myself hitting the ground and not having to think about my life anymore. I also thought about the potential regret I may feel when I first took the leap. It scared me a bit that I wouldn't be able to take it back once I stepped off. I had to put more thought into it. I went back inside and sat on the edge of my bed. I tried to rationally think about if it was worth it to continue living. I knew I could eventually sort out my financial issues once I became a pharmacist and worked for a few years. That was solvable. There was no way for me to prevent people from thinking I was crazy. This is something I would have to live with. I had to go from the military pharmacist who travelled the world playing basketball to a mentally ill civilian who made it clear on social media he was crazy. I wasn't sure I could live with this. If I knew at the time how poorly I would be treated in the future by the military and Nova Scotia College of Pharmacists because of my illness, I would have cut the net and jumped with no regret. Luckily, I was blind to how powerful the mental health stigma really is.

After spending some time thinking about my options. I concluded that I had no will to live, but I was too scared to actually go through with killing myself. I remembered the pain my family experienced when my mother passed away and I couldn't put them through that again. I had to figure something out. I decided to fight through my embarrassment and call my sister. Luckily, she was off that day and she answered the phone right away. Once I heard her voice, I instantly cried. I told her the truth. I told her I was thinking about killing myself.

My sister is really good at taking control of situations like this. She instantly got stern with me. "Listen, Garrett. We were waiting for this to happen and it's completely normal with Bipolar. You must get dressed, get in your car, and drive to the base. Don't hold anything back. Tell them you're having suicidal thoughts. They'll know what to do." I told her I would. It was a struggle to dress myself. I was starving and had no energy to move. I left my apartment, made my way down the hall to the elevator, and travelled down to the parking garage. Once I got to my vehicle, I instantly cried again. I felt completely miserable. I started the car and drove to the base.

When I pulled up to the clinic, I couldn't get myself to get out of the car. I didn't want all of the people I worked with to see me in such a vulnerable state. I knew I needed help, but my body wouldn't let me open the car door. I was frozen. I continued to sob and tears kept rolling down my face. I felt at that moment it would be easier for me to be dead.

I thought nothing would ever get better. I called my sister back and told her I was in the parking lot, but I couldn't go in. She stopped me when I tried to reason with her. "Garrett. I will stay on the phone with you. Open the car door right now and get out of the car," she pleaded with me. I listened to her instructions. She then told me to walk towards the clinic and open the door. She stayed on the phone with me right until I got to the reception area. I hung up and lifted my head to the receptionist. "I need to talk to someone," I said.

She could see I had just cried when she looked at me. She asked for my service number and looked up my record. A nurse came out from behind the counter and brought me to a waiting area in a hallway around the corner. I sat there for about ten minutes, waiting to get into a treatment room. People I worked with kept walking by and saying hello. I was completely broken but tried my hardest to fake a smile and say hello back to them. I just wanted to be alone and out of sight. A physician eventually opened the door to her office and invited me in. We talked for a little while and then, after establishing my diagnosis and the fact that I was clearly experiencing severe depression, she thought it would be best for me to speak to my psychiatrist. She made a phone call to Dr. Edwards and he informed her he had just finished with an appointment and could see me immediately. We exited her office and made our way up to the mental health unit. I entered his office and sat on the couch. This time I was in a different state. He could tell I was struggling. We talked for a little while about what I was thinking. I eventually told him I feared the thoughts I was having. I admitted to him I was having suicidal thoughts. He asked if I wanted to be admitted, but I really didn't want to go back to a hospital. I told him I could probably contact Hannah and let her know what's going on. I could stay with her. He agreed that he would let me go if I was accompanied by someone. He didn't want me going back to my apartment alone.

After we had a plan in place, we moved on to discuss treatment options. He felt it would be best to give me an antidepressant and chose sertraline as it would have less of a chance to push me back into mania. I agreed that I needed something to get me through this rough patch and gladly accepted the medication. He then told me that he will do everything he can to get me in to speak with the psychologist as soon as possible.

After we finished our conversation, he had me contact Hannah to make sure I had someone to look after me. Luckily, she answered, and there were no issues. I was relieved that I didn't have to go back to the hospital. I left the office and made my way to the pharmacy to get another prescription filled. It was embarrassing for me to let them all know I was clinically depressed by handing in the prescription, but I knew I needed the medication. I was scared to death I had no desire to live. I was scared I would take my own life if I didn't get something to help. They got the prescription ready right away and I was on my way home.

Once I got in the car, I called Hannah again. I put the phone on speaker and asked if I could talk to her on the way home. She agreed and stayed on the phone with me the whole time. She came over to meet me as I pulled up to my building and helped me up to my apartment. Once we walked in the door, I broke down again. I was so overwhelmed by the day. I cried like a baby as I hugged Hannah. I explained to her I didn't know what was happening to me. She placed her hands on my face and told me it would be okay. She said that we would get through this together. I really wanted to believe her, but I couldn't get past the darkness of my thoughts. She helped me pack a bag and we made our way over to her apartment. I hung out in her bedroom while she made me some food.

I stayed at her apartment for a few weeks, just going back to my apartment to get new clothes. Eventually, the medication kicked in and I became able to make my own food and get myself out of bed in the morning. Throughout these first few weeks, I also had a couple of appointments with the psychologist. We talked for an hour each session and worked our way to the root of my issue. I didn't want to accept that I had Bipolar Disorder. I didn't want to leave the military; it meant a lot to be a part of the organization. Lastly, I didn't want everyone to look at me as someone who is mentally ill. I just wanted to be my confident self and a pharmacy officer after working so hard to achieve it. She worked with me a lot to gain acceptance of the situation but deep down, I still had myself convinced that I didn't have bipolar. I had a mental breakdown and that was the end of it for me.

Things got better over the next few months, and I was invited to play for the military's national basketball team in Belgium in December. Typically, I wouldn't be able to go on the trip because I was on a medical category, but my psychiatrist wrote me a letter saying he thought it would be good for my mental health to attend. We trained in Ottawa for a week then flew to Belgium for a tournament.

During my time in Belgium, I felt completely back to normal. I was in my element. I was hanging out with a great group of guys and playing the sport I loved. I was simply enjoying life. One night after our second game, I was in the bathroom after showering. It was time to take my medication, but I was hesitant. I thought to myself that since I'm doing so well, I probably don't really need them anymore. It has been a few months since my mental breakdown, and I wasn't feeling depressed. Most of all, I just wanted to be like the rest of the guys. I didn't want to rely on medication to get through life. I looked at myself in the mirror and told myself that I can handle this. I put my medication back in my bag, got dressed, and went to join the guys. I had a great time during the rest of the trip and we soon headed back to Canada.

When I landed back in Halifax, I had a renewed sense of self. I was proud of myself for coming off my medication and felt like a normal person again. It made me feel like I was stronger for not needing them. I was honest with Hannah and my psychiatrist when I saw them next. I didn't try to hide it from them. My psychiatrist warned me it wasn't a good idea but said that the decision was mine to make. He told me to watch out for signs of my mood changing and decided that we would see each other a little more often.

Over the next few months, there were no hiccups. I continued to have frequent visits with the psychologist and psychiatrist and studied hard for my licensing exam coming up in May. I worked in the base pharmacy daily and once a week, I would give a presentation on whichever topic I was studying. Everything in my life seemed back on track. I was still upset I would be released from the military, but I had grown to have a bit more acceptance of the situation. I tried to focus on the positive side of it and be happy that I would most likely get to move back to Sydney sooner than expected to be near my family.

I wrote my exam in May and felt very confident about it. All of the hard work I had put in over the months leading to it seemed to have paid off. To make matters even better, Hannah and I moved into an apartment together near the base. Just two months later, it was July and I got my results. I had passed. I was finally back on track with my career and was a licensed pharmacist in the matter of a couple of short weeks. I was finally able to check prescriptions in the pharmacy and was soon given the responsibility of second in command at work. Unfortunately, this is when I got into trouble mentally.

I was told by my superiors at the base that because I was on a medical category, they could not promote me to Captain. It would take another year for the release process to go through, so this meant that I would have to work for a full year getting paid about $20,000 less than my peers based solely on my having a mental illness. I had a really hard time handling this news. I thought about everything we learned in school about the stigma attached to mental illness and how it's not right to treat people unfairly due to their illness. I thought about the Bell Let's Talk campaign and how everyone seemingly comes together every year to treat people with respect when they suffer from an illness. It didn't seem fair to me. I tried to talk with my immediate supervisor about the issue a couple of times and he said that the best he could do would be to try and get me a payment after I was released. This would never happen. I spoke with another Captain I was close with and he instructed me to talk to a lawyer. He made it abundantly clear that if they have me working for them as a pharmacist, I should be paid as a pharmacist. I agreed and got very upset about the situation.

My anger towards the situation made me feel very driven. I tried speaking with my chain of command, but they also said that they couldn't help me. One of my coworkers told me I should be grateful for everything the military has done for me and let it go. This only made me feel more upset. How could I be thankful to an organization that's telling me I'm not good enough to remain in it?

After coming to grips with the fact that I wasn't not going to be paid a pharmacist's salary, I thought of ways I could make up the difference. I was still in debt from my time in school and the previous summer I had with Arbonne during my first manic episode. I considered giving Arbonne another try. Little did I know, I was slowly becoming manic again and the risky business idea was a symptom of my hypomania. The stress of getting treated differently due to my diagnosis was too much for me.

I started by talking with Hannah about Arbonne and telling her it would be a great thing for both of us to do together. I acknowledged that things got a little out of hand last time but told her that I was better now and was ready to give it a real try. She was hesitant at first, but I continued to press her until she agreed with me. We contacted the NVP from the previous summer and told her we both wanted to sign up. We met with her a few days later and placed two orders for $1000 each. A couple of days later, we had a launch party and a few of Hannah's friends signed up. We quickly had a small team assembled and were ready to expand.

A couple of days later while I was working at the pharmacy, I had a patient come to the counter and talk about the issues he was going through while he was waiting for his prescription. He talked about how he was waiting to get medically released and was pissed off at the way the military was treating him. He told me he didn't know what he would do after he got out; he had no skills that could transfer to the real world. I really felt bad for him as I was going through a similar situation. I saw him at the gym later that day and approached him. I told him about the business I recently got into and told him to call me if he ever wanted to discuss it. I mentioned that I could take him out to eat and explain what it's all about. I really thought that I was doing the right thing and trying to help him. I was proud of myself for reaching out. We decided that we would meet in a couple of days on the weekend and I gave him my number. This happened on a Tuesday.

When I got home that day, I felt a surge in energy. I thought of different ways I could speed up getting our team built. I made a Facebook group for our small team and recorded a video message to the group explaining the purpose of it. After posting my video, I decided that I would try to do a daily video to keep the group motivated. I stayed on my computer for hours thinking of ideas to grow the business. Hannah eventually came into the computer room and told me she was going to bed. I knew she would try to stop me if I said I wanted to stay up; she was really on top of my sleeping habits since my first episode. I decided to lay in bed until she fell asleep and then got back up to work. While I was on the computer, I had a sudden urge to smoke cannabis. I remembered the way it made me feel during the last summer when I was manic, and I wanted that same feeling. I wanted to experience the abilities again.

I texted a friend I knew from school and he agreed to deliver some. I had it within 30 minutes. I grabbed a pair of scissors and went into the computer room to roll a joint. After it was done, I brought it out onto the balcony to smoke it. I lit it with my barbeque lighter and once I took my first puff, I could feel my abilities coming back. I felt powerful. I stood in a power pose facing the base and thought about how they were treating me unfairly due to having a mental illness. I wanted to get paid the same as the other pharmacists. I thought about how wrong it was. I was obsessed.

With each puff, my powers grew. I had anxiety that the police would sense I was back and that they would come to stop me again. I thought back to my first time feeling this way and realized that I had to keep this to myself or I would end up in the hospital again. I couldn't let that happen. I needed to reach my goals this time. I threw the joint and went inside. When I stepped in, I closed my eyes and took a deep breath. I had to get myself under control. I recalled that last time, I stopped eating. I went to the kitchen and made myself some food. I brought it over the living area and sat on the couch. When I turned on the TV, The Matrix was playing. I had an epiphany. The television was showing me the truth about my reality. I was living in the Matrix the whole time and I didn't realize it until that moment. I finally understood that every time I left my apartment, I was in the matrix and anything was possible. It was up to me, however, to make it happen. I smiled and felt excitement rushing through my body.

When I finished eating, I went back into the computer room. I put on my headphones and played some rap songs with the volume turned all the way up. I realized right away that the songs were made for me and that they were speaking direct messages. I listened to each song so intently to make sure I didn't miss out on the intended message. I felt so powerful listening to what they had wrote for me. I soon recalled that during my first experience with my powers, I didn't sleep much so I should try to correct it. I shut off the music and went into the bedroom. Hannah was sound asleep, so I snuck in the bed next to her. I laid there with my eyes closed but didn't fall asleep. I thought about how I would work hard to make this time different. I wouldn't allow myself to lose control and force my family to call the police on me.

I stayed in bed until my alarm clock went off. I got up, shaved, showered, and put on my uniform. I ate some breakfast then headed down to the base for my shift. My energy didn't feel as high, but I knew I still had to be cautious. I didn't socialize as much as I usually do at work. I just did my job and tried to fly under the radar. During my lunch break, I thought about how good it would feel when my Arbonne business grew and I could prove to my family I wasn't crazy after all. I thought I should get ready for the money to roll in by creating a business account at a bank. I unlocked my phone and called the closest Scotiabank to my location. When they answered, I told them I needed to set up and business account and asked when their next appointment was. They asked if I was available this afternoon and I said yes without hesitation. I hung up the phone and walked over to my team lead's office. I asked him if I could step out for an appointment at the bank and he gave me the nod.

I walked to my apartment and got into my car. I drove to the bank, parked, and stepped inside. I was walking in with my head held high. They would soon know me as the guy with the lucrative business. I told the receptionist I was here for an appointment to set up a business account. She directed me towards an office nearby and said he is ready for me in there. I walked over and the man met me outside, shook my hand and invited me in. He started by asking me what type of business I was going to using the account for. I told him it was a network marketing company and that it was only small now, but I felt like it would grow rather quickly. I told him that because I already had a salary with my work as a pharmacist, I wanted to invest the money in stocks. We talked a bit about it and he said that once the money comes in that we can open up an eTrade account to buy and sell stocks. I was getting excited by the thought of it.

The appointment didn't last long as it was a pretty simple process. As it was winding down, I told him I would probably need a business credit card as well. He told me to just hang on for a moment and he would see if his coworker was available. They both showed up back in the office and the new guy asked me to come with him. I followed him downstairs to his office and we talked about all of the credit cards they offered. I told him about the business and asked him to pick whichever card he thought was best. I wasn't too picky about which credit card I got and I trusted his judgement. We filled out the paperwork and he told me I should get my card in the mail in five to ten business days. I shook his hand and made my way out of the bank. I felt like it was a very pleasant experience and I looked forward to working with them in the future.

I didn't bother going back to work after my time at the bank. I just went straight home. When I entered my apartment, I changed my clothes and went right into the computer room to make a motivational video for the team. I had extra high energy and was much more enthusiastic in this video. After I finished, I got a text from the military member I was speaking with at the gym the other day. He said he wanted to meet up to discuss the business. I was elated. I felt like everything would finally start to fall into place. I told him we would meet up that night. With a sudden burst of energy, I felt the urge to smoke some cannabis. I felt like I needed the added energy it would give me. I rolled a joint and went for a walk to a nearby park. I stood in the open field and smoked.

Just like the night before, my mind instantly produced irregular thoughts. I focused hard on the fact that the military wasn't paying me a pharmacist's wage and thought about my coworker telling me I should get a lawyer. I decided that it was important and had to happen that day. I would call my friend, Markus, once I got back home. I had a renewed sense of power take over when I made that decision. I recalled my discovery from the night before that I was living in the Matrix and could do anything I wanted while out in the world. I thought I should get some accessories for my meeting with my soon to be team member. I finished smoking the joint and walked back to my apartment. I went right down into the underground parking and got into my car. I drove to Staples just down the road.

I went inside and asked the first worker I saw to direct me to the briefcases. They pointed me to the back portion of the store. When I arrived in the right section, I liked what I saw. One briefcase stood out from the others. It was Bugatti brand. I needed it. There were some black umbrellas next to the briefcases. I grabbed one and examined it. It was perfect. The briefcase and umbrella were perfect accessories to bring into the Matrix with me. I brought them up to the counter and paid. I can recall being upset I didn't yet have my business credit card.

I left with my items and headed home. When I walked into my apartment, I instantly put everything down and called my friend, who was a lawyer. He picked up and I instantly explained the situation to him. I told him that the military was underpaying me based on having a mental illness and that it wasn't right. I explained that I wanted to put them in their place for treating me so horribly. I asked him how I could know he was my lawyer and told him I wanted to send him a retainer. He ensured me he would help me if I wanted to pursue something but told me it wasn't necessary to send him money at that time. I wouldn't take no for an answer. In my mind, I was alone against the military unless he took money from me. He could sense I would not give up and told me he would put me through to his receptionist and bill me $500 dollars as a retainer if it would make me feel better. I was instantly thankful. Now I felt like Markus was on my team and had my back.

After I hung up with him, Hannah was getting home from school. I met her at the door and told her all about my day. I told her I went to the bank to open a business account, set up an Arbonne meeting for tonight, hired Markus as my lawyer, and went shopping at Staples. I pointed towards my briefcase. She had a concerned look on her face. "Garrett, are you feeling ok?" she asked. I told her I felt great and was just excited that I got so much done today. She continued to tell me she thought I was speaking really fast and that I seemed to have a lot of energy. She recommended calling my sister to check in with her and explain how I feel.

I became really upset with Hannah. I tried hard to resist from raising my voice. I promised her I was okay and didn't feel comfortable calling my sister after what she did last summer. She ruined my business once and I would not let her ruin it again. I told her not to get concerned every time I'm happy. I explained to her I was allowed to be happy sometimes and it doesn't mean there's an issue. She was persistent with me. She said I never shop for myself, I already told her I wasn't going to get a lawyer, and that I didn't need a business account yet. All of this seemed out of character to her. I felt like I was under the microscope and it really pissed me off. My head started to spin. I finally raised my voice. "Stop acting like you understand me! I'm allowed to enjoy my life! If you want to understand what's going on, watch the movie The Matrix! All the answers are in it!" I turned around, grabbed my briefcase and went into the computer room. I slammed the door behind me. I felt some anxiety. I didn't know if it was a smart idea to tell Hannah about the matrix. I didn't know if she could handle the truth.

I spent some time alone in the computer room and then eventually texted the guy I met at the gym. I asked him if he wanted to pick me up in a cab around 7:00 pm so we could head downtown. I told him I would pay for everything. He agreed. I went back out into the main living area and Hannah was just opening the door for friend, Martha. She was on our Arbonne team and was one of Hannah's best friends. I said hello but quickly walked by them and into the bathroom. I took a long shower and when I came back out, I noticed that Hannah and Martha were watching The Matrix movie. I thought to myself how crazy it would be when they realized that the truth was right in front of them all this time.

I texted my new friend to tell him he can leave anytime and I went into the bedroom to get dressed. I wore jeans with a blazer and a white t-shirt underneath. I came back out into the main area, put my shoes on and brought my briefcase into the computer room to load it up. I didn't want to waste too much time explaining the whole business plan to him, so I brought items to represent the plan and some books he could read on his own time to help him understand. I grabbed a book about investing called The Lazy Investor and a network marketing book called Go Pro. I threw them into my briefcase. I then noticed my hourglass sitting on the desk. I placed it in my briefcase as well. I grabbed random items and placing them all in the briefcase. Everything from a portable cell phone charger to my passport. When I felt like it was sufficiently packed. I left the room.

Hannah instantly got up off the couch and approached me as I entered the main area. She put her hands on my face and told me she would feel a lot better if I stayed home tonight. I told her she need not be scared and to finish watching the movie. I said that I know what I'm doing and she'll understand after she finishes it. She looked really concerned. She was scared that I was turning manic, but I interpreted it as her being scared that I was going out into the matrix. Devon stood up off the couch and tried to help Hannah. "Why don't you just tell the guy you're meeting to come over here?" she asked. I told them both I was 100% going on this meeting and that they had to calm down. We were just going to a restaurant to talk. I shrugged off Hannah as I felt my phone buzz in my pocket. "I'm almost there," read the text. I grabbed my umbrella and briefcase and went outside to wait for the taxi. Once I stepped outside the front door to the building, I was in the matrix. Anything was possible.

It was lightly raining so when the taxi pulled up, I had my umbrella open overhead and was holding my briefcase base by my side. I got into the back seat and shook his hand. His name was Evan. I told him I know a great spot that's really private. It would be a great place for us to chat. I asked the taxi driver to take us to The Middle Spoon. When he pulled up, the green cactus-shaped light in the window was on, so the secret restaurant in the basement was open. I walked inside with Evan and said the password to one waitress. "Right this way," she responded. We followed her down the stairs by the back wall and through the kitchen in the basement. We walked down a long hallway and after she explained the rules to us, we entered Noble. I got a table in the back corner. The music and décor were out of the 30s during prohibition times. It was a dimly lit lounge area with only about 20 guests. I truly felt like I was playing the matrix like a fiddle. I was in the perfect spot doing exactly what I wanted to be doing.

I lifted my briefcase to the table opened it up. I explained to Evan that everything we needed to make money was right here. We talked for a little while about the plan of making money through Arbonne and dumping it all into dividend stocks to build a portfolio for the long term. I told him that if he read these two books, he would completely understand how we would make money and then have that money work for us for the rest of our lives. Just as he started to ask questions, the waitress approached the table. I quickly closed the briefcase. I couldn't let her see what we were talking about. "Aren't you mysterious," she said. She continued to ask us what we'd like to order. I reminded Evan he could have whatever he'd like. I ordered a Penicillin for my drink. It was a lemon-flavored whiskey cocktail. I also ordered a piece of a peanut butter cheesecake. I felt like because I was in the matrix, I could live it up and enjoy anything I wanted. Evan ordered a cocktail but said he didn't need any food. I assumed that he didn't fully comprehend the situation. He must not have understood that once you acknowledge you're in the matrix, you can live like a king.

The waitress left the table, and we continued our discussion. We talked for ten minutes about Arbonne, and then I told him I didn't want to waste the entire evening discussing my plan. I told him he could take the information I gave him and think about it until he's ready to decide. Our order came and it was time to enjoy the night. I put everything away, closed my briefcase, and set it on the ground beside the table. We discussed our situation with the military and he was still pretty upset about it. I put a positive spin on everything telling him it would free up more time for us to grow the business and give us more personal freedom. I could see that while we were talking, he was eyeing my cheesecake. I got up from the table and went to get a second fork, I came back to the table and handed it to him. I told him to take a bite and enjoy himself. He was hesitant at first. He said it's not really his thing to share a desert with another guy. I told him to let go of his insecurity and take a fucking bite. He stuck his fork into the cake, lifted it to his mouth and I could see him perk up. "How good is that?" I asked. "It's pretty fucking delicious," he replied. We both continued to shovel it into our mouths until it was gone. I raised my hand to the waitress and asked for my bill. I paid shortly after and we exited the bar onto a side street.

I called a cab and then told him we should keep the night going. I asked him what his favorite food was and he told me it was steak. I suggested we go buy two T-bone steaks and bring them to my place to barbecue. Evan thought it was a pretty good idea. I called a cab and we drove to a nearby grocery store. Once we bought the steaks, I couldn't help myself but to post on social media. I set my status to "10 pm steak night." I felt like I had to brag about how perfect my life was and how much fun I was having. This would be my life every day going forward.

We made it back to my apartment and Hannah was still up waiting for me. She said nothing to me about my symptoms of mania because I had a guest with me. I offered Evan a drink, made myself a martini, and fired up the barbecue. Evan told me all about his dream of becoming a chef, so I let him take the reins on the grill. I told him to show me what he can do. I was feeling pretty pumped up and I knew it was time to take things to another level. I rushed into the computer room and quickly rolled a joint. I brought it out onto the patio and lit it up. I stood in a power pose while I smoked it staring down the street at the base. I fixated again on how the military was treating me differently than my coworkers because of my diagnosis. I could feel myself getting angry, so I tried to shut it out of my mind.

As I continued to smoke the joint, I developed some anxiety. I was worried that the creators of the matrix were tracking me and knew that I had figured it all out. They knew that I could bring the whole system down if I woke up enough people to the truth. I felt threatened. I knew I had to be more careful and not flaunt that I knew what reality really was.

Evan finished cooking the steaks, so we went inside to eat. I locked the door behind me as I entered the apartment. While we ate, I told him about how big of an opportunity we have to help people. Once we build up a good amount of wealth, we can help people like us that are struggling getting released from the military. We can help anyone we like once we put in the work and get to where we need to be. He agreed that it would be nice to be able to do that but still felt like he needed some time to think about the opportunity and if it was right for him. He stayed for another hour or so and then was ready to head home. I called him a cab and gave them my credit card information for them to charge me.

When he was ready to leave, I became anxious again. I was nervous that the controllers of the matrix would send someone to harm Evan. I felt like they knew that we were living outside of the normal rules and that we might be in trouble. We were enjoying ourselves a little too much. I walked out into the lobby with him and made sure that we stood in front of the security camera while we waited. This way no one could harm us. It would all be on video if they tried to do something. I felt a little more at ease. When the cab showed up, my anxiety spiked again. Evan left through the front doors of the lobby. What if he gets shot? What if someone approaches him and kills him? All of these thoughts rushed through my mind. I just wanted him to make it to the cab alive. He walked down the steps and reached for the car door. "Come on. Get in," I thought. He opened the door and got inside. The cab pulled away. I turned around and stared into the security camera. I was staring at the controllers. I felt like I had won because Evan made it away safely.

I went back into the apartment and Hannah approached me to ask how I was feeling. I told her I was feeling great and was pumped up over

Evan being most likely going to sign with us. She asked if I was ready for bed and reminded me I have work in the morning. I really wasn't tired, but I knew I had to go to bed with her or this conversation would never end. I got undressed, brushed my teeth, and made my way to bed. I couldn't sleep. I spent most of the night planning how I would sign more members to our team and how I could get our current team members more active. I was a bit frustrated that no one seemed to want to work as much as I did. I eventually dozed off for a couple of hours and then woke up to my alarm clock. I went through my morning routine and left to go to work.

When I arrived at work, I felt myself obsess over my pay again. I couldn't let go of my diagnosis being held against me and that I was being treated differently than my coworkers. I really needed the extra money after my first episode and I was so sure I would get it after becoming a pharmacist. Instead, nothing changed. I was just given more responsibility with no financial benefit. It was really weighing on my mind. Around nine o'clock, I left the pharmacy and went up to the mental health unit for an appointment with my psychiatrist. It didn't take me long to fill him in on how I felt about the whole situation. I tried to explain it all to him, but halfway through, I broke down into tears. I was just so frustrated. It made me feel like I was below everyone else. I was doing the exact same work but being treated differently all because of a medical label given to me. I couldn't handle it.

It took me a little while to gather myself and stop the tears. Dr. Edwards said he thought it would be best to give me a couple of days off of work to relax and get myself together. He handed me a form to give to my team lead and I left the office. He didn't suspect that mania was coming through; I didn't really give him a reason to think anything was wrong. I probably looked more depressed than manic. Maybe I should have told him about my thoughts of being in the matrix. It would have been a good opportunity to get help. I thought it was the truth, though, and that he wouldn't believe me. There was no point in explaining the truth of our reality to him.

It felt good to leave the base. I didn't like being in a place that made me feel inferior – especially for medical reasons. I was extra careful walking home. I didn't want the controllers to see me acting happy. I made sure to follow the rules. I only crossed the street at crosswalks and stuck to the right side of the sidewalk to get home. I did nothing to stand out. When I made it home to my apartment, I took a deep breath and a sigh of relief. I felt like I was lucky to have made it back safely.

I had a lot of energy, but I was still feeling a bit down emotionally so I rolled a joint to help me level up a bit. I wanted to feel like I felt the night before. I wanted more ideas to rush into my mind. I had the whole day to myself since Hannah was at school, so I figured it was a good day to get a lot done.

I went to the computer room to roll a joint, then got dressed, left my apartment, and walked up to the nearby park. I lit the joint and again, with the first puff, I felt my powers come back. I felt strong. I felt like I had special abilities again. Ideas flowed forward into my mind just like I had hoped. With each puff, my powers grew. I felt like I was an infinite human again just like the summer of 2014. It felt incredible. I finished the joint and threw it on the ground. Walking back to my apartment, I wasn't scared. I didn't fear the controllers anymore. I felt like I was in control and they were scrambling to regain it. Humans weren't supposed to get this strong in the matrix. They were supposed to stay grounded. I could break the matrix if I wanted to. I could kill the controllers. I didn't want to be violent, though. I only wanted to live my life and enjoy myself. I wanted to put in some work and get the results out of life that have been denied to me.

When I got back to my building, I put my hand on the door to enter the lobby but then realized that I didn't have to hide in my apartment. I should be enjoying myself. I turned around and took in my surroundings. I looked at the bakery across the street. I thought it would be a perfect place to grab a snack. I walked across the street ignoring crosswalks and sidewalks. I went straight for the door. When I stepped inside, I scanned everyone. I wanted to make sure there were no controllers inside. Everything seemed ok. I walked up to the cashier and asked her to give me a coffee and her most popular two deserts. She came back with a fruit trifle and a chocolate cake. It was perfect. I brought it to a table and slowly ate it. I moaned with every bite. It was delicious. I loved being in the matrix. Whatever I wanted was mine. I knew I would have to leave it someday now that I knew the truth, but while I was here, I wanted to explore and enjoy what it offered.

After I finished, I looked up the bakery on Facebook and liked their page. That was how I would leave my mark and show my support for the businesses that were good to me. I was doing them a huge favor by associating my name with them. I exited the bakery and went down to the next store on the strip. It was a sushi restaurant. I went inside and sat down. When the waitress came over to hand me a menu, I said, "Two spicy tuna rolls and a Stella Artois." It took about 10 minutes for it to arrive. Again, I couldn't help but moan with each bite. Everything tasted so real. I was impressed at how sophisticated the matrix had become. When I finished eating, I tipped the waitress 50%. I knew that generosity went a long way in this place. I took my last sip of beer and left the restaurant.

I decided that I had enough fun, and it was time to head home and get back to work. I walked across the street to my building. Once I got inside my apartment, I took off my shoes and jacket and went straight into the computer room. I sat down and really thought about what I wanted to be. I knew I was already a pharmacist and about to be an NVP for Arbonne, but I wanted more. I knew that I could be anything. Whatever I thought of, the matrix would deliver. I decided I wanted to be a rapper. I could represent my island by doing performances around the world. I reached into the filing cabinet next to the computer desk and took out a note pad. I wrote down my first rap line by line. It was coming effortlessly. I wrote down lines about my family, past relationships, and the military. It took me about an hour to get my first song completed. I turned on my webcam and recorded it with no background music. It was just me and the camera. After I finished recording, I went to Facebook to post it. As I was watching it upload, I thought of my family stopping me from doing what I wanted the previous summer. I felt threatened that they would come to stop me again if they saw this song. I cancelled the upload. I would wait for a better time to post it.

After my rap session, I pressed record on the Arbonne Facebook group and sent a video message out to my team for motivation. It was a quick message as I was probably talking a mile a minute. I imagined my team getting the message and quickly going out to sign multiple consultants and clients. I could feel the white Mercedes manifesting into my life. I wanted to put more time into Arbonne, but I felt like I had bigger things going on.

I realized soon after that, I hadn't yet told Hannah about my appointment. I was thinking she would be happy now that we'd be able to spend more time together since I wasn't working. I called her but she didn't answer. I assumed she was busy in class, so I sent her a heartfelt text. I explained the situation and told her how much I loved her. She replied thanking me for letting her know and that she'd be home soon. I cleaned the apartment so she'd be in a good mood when she returned. I didn't think I had much time so I rushed through it. I tidied the living area, cleaned the kitchen, swept the floor, and made our bed. She got home just as I was finishing.

Once she walked in, I ran over to give her a hug. I told her I wanted to take her out to eat so we can get some sushi. I filled her in that I went to the sushi place across the street and told her how incredible it was. She kind of laughed at how excited I was and agreed that I could take her out. I was so excited. It would be the first time I took Hannah out into the matrix with me. I was a little bit nervous, but I figured that the controllers knew not to mess with me. They had seen what I'm capable of. I knew that I would have to be on high alert, but I was confident I could protect her.

Hannah went in through the bedroom to grab a shower, so I ran to the computer room to roll another joint. I brought it up to the park and lit it. I needed more power so I could adequately protect Hannah when I brought her out with me. Every puff made me feel more and more powerful yet again. I could now think clearly. I could see everything that I had to do to reach my goals. I would make tonight a big night after Hannah went to bed. I didn't have work in the morning, so there was no reason for me to sleep. I was excited to see what else I could accomplish.

I left the park and went back into my apartment. Hannah was out of the shower and asked me where I went. I told her I went to the park to smoke a joint, and she said that it's probably not a good idea for me to be smoking so much weed. She mentioned that she noticed I had been doing it too often the last few days. I told her I was just stressed and needed it to relax a bit. I ensured her I wouldn't make a habit out of it. I did not ease her stress, but we moved on from the conversation. I told her I was really excited to take her out and she went back to getting ready.

I used the time while she was getting ready to jump back onto my computer. I checked how many views my motivational video received to get an idea if people were actually watching them and listened to my rap a couple of times. I wanted to stay home and write another one, but I committed to going out so I knew I should stick with the original plan. While I was on Facebook, the computer screen flashed. I took it as a sign that someone working at Facebook was trying to give me a signal. What were they trying to say? This really made me want to spend more time on the computer, but Hannah called. She was ready to go. I would come back to Facebook later in the evening and figure out what the message was supposed to mean.

I got up from the desk and went out to meet Hannah. We put on our shoes and jackets and left the apartment. Once we walked outside, I had a bit of anxiety surface. I knew Hannah was in danger being with me, but I also knew I had the power to protect her. I scanned everyone we passed on the sidewalk as we walked to the restaurant. I made sure to have my hands out of my pockets in case I had to engage in a physical altercation. I was ready if it happened. I wasn't too concerned about girls we passed, but every guy was a threat. I didn't know who was a controller and who wasn't. Were they just watching me or did they have a plan to get us at some point during the evening? I was ready and willing to kill someone if they tried to attack us. I would let no one get near Hannah.

We made it to the restaurant and went inside to take a seat. I made it clear to Hannah she could get whatever she wanted and then excused myself to go to the bathroom. When I got inside, I splashed some water on my face and stared at myself in the mirror. I was looking directly into my eyes and widening them with intense focus. I looked at my hands and could feel my power. I knew that anything was possible in the matrix, but I questioned just how powerful I was. Did I have superhuman strength? Was I able to fly? Could I at least levitate? Would I be able to read minds? I didn't know what the future had in store for me, but I looked forward to experiencing it. I used the bathroom, washed my hands, and went back to Hannah.

We got a bunch of different types of rolls and a bottle of wine. I loved being there with her. I was happy that I took her deep into the matrix with me. Each time I looked at her, I felt like we could conquer the world. Our food eventually came and we enjoyed every bite. It was washed down with the wine. We spent some time talking after we finished and eventually paid and left to head home. I was excited the whole way home to try and figure out what message Facebook was trying to send me before we left for our date.

When we arrived back home, Hannah wanted to hang out for a little while before bed. I really wanted to go right into the computer room, but I stayed with her in the living room to watch some television. It was hard to keep my composure during commercial breaks because I knew that each commercial was designed for me and that they were sending me messages. Hannah had no idea and I knew I couldn't tell her about my discovery. I didn't want to scare her. Each time a product was advertised I took it as an instruction to purchase the item. It wasn't just a recommendation; it was an order. I tried to mentally note each item displayed to me but eventually, there were too many to keep track of. We hung out for about an hour and then Hannah wanted to get in bed. I would have to do my normal routine and wait until she fell asleep to get my work done.

The wine helped Hannah fall asleep quickly and then I snuck out of the bed. I went into the computer room, rolled a joint, and brought it out onto the balcony. After I finished smoking, I went right to work. I went onto the computer and logged into Facebook. I kept clicking different buttons trying to get the signal from them. Eventually the screen flashed again and a pop-up appeared asking me to fill out a survey. I knew this was no ordinary survey. This was an application to work for Facebook. I was amazed. Finally, I was getting some recognition for everything I was doing. I took my time filling out the survey and answered every question with care. It took a long time to fill out, but I was relishing in the fact that Facebook wanted to hire me. Everyone in my family would be so proud of me. People would wonder how a guy from Cape Breton got hired to work for one of the tech giants. Sadly, I could never tell them the truth of how it all happened.

After I finished the application, I grabbed my headphones and plugged them into my phone. I played rap music on max volume and went out onto the balcony. I stood outside, looking down at the base. I stood in a power pose. I thought about how sorry the military would be for kicking me out. They would wish they let me stay in the organization after seeing everything that I accomplished. They would wish they paid me a fair wage and didn't ruin the respect I had for them. I thought to myself about how good of a captain I would have been. I felt emotional. I knew deep down I didn't want to leave the Canadian Forces, but at least I was moving on to bigger things. Then it dawned on me.

Since Facebook hired me in such a secretive way, I knew that I had to hide all of the proof of what happened. I ran off the balcony and into the kitchen. I rummaged through the drawers and grabbed all of the plastic bags I could find of every size. I brought them into the computer room. I had to clean up all of the evidence. Anything with my fingerprints on it would have to go. I grabbed anything that I touched and placed each item into its own plastic bag. I grabbed pens, books, decorations, even my computer mouse. Each item had to have its own bag. I pilled everything in the middle of the room. It took me over an hour to gather everything up. Every book off of my bookshelf was now sealed in a zip lock bag and sitting on the floor.

I ran to another room and grabbed a plastic tote. I threw the bagged items into the tote and then put on the lid. It was a clear plastic so you could still see the items. I quickly went into the kitchen and gathered two black garbage bags. I brought them into the room and put them over the tote on opposite sides. The items were finally hidden. I put the tote into the closet and closed the door. When I turned around, I realized that the computer itself was evidence of what I was doing. I ripped it apart. I opened the closet door and threw in the keyboard, the speakers, the monitor and then the CPU. I went back into the kitchen and grabbed a cloth and ran it under water. I hurried back into the computer room and wiped down my desk. After I was finished, I wiped down the walls and door of the closet. I was finally done.

I realized quickly that Mark Zuckerberg of Facebook would want to meet me. I assumed that they would send a car to pick me up and bring me to the airport. Now that everything was hidden, they would most likely come the next morning. I grabbed my briefcase and placed it on the kitchen counter. I snuck into the bedroom and grabbed a change of clothes. I put them in the briefcase. Next, I found my passport and put it in as well. I gathered my driver's license and military ID. I knew I wouldn't need my debit of credit card as everything on this trip would be paid for. Once my briefcase was packed, I put it down on the floor next to the front door of the apartment. I got a shower in our second bathroom and put on some nice clothes. I was ready.

I spent most of the night going back and forth from the balcony to smoke joints and the living room to watch commercials and make a note of what items I was supposed to purchase. I stayed up all night. When the morning came around and the sun was rising. I grabbed my briefcase and went out onto the front step. I sat down and waited for my ride to come and pick me up. I sat there for about two hours and still no one had shown up. I thought that maybe I hadn't hidden the items in the plastic tote good enough. Surely if I had, I would have already been on a plane. I needed to find a secure place to put the tote. I thought that maybe the bank would be a good spot if they had large enough safety deposit boxes. I went back inside.

When I opened the door to the apartment, Hannah was awake and got out of bed. She asked me what I was doing up so early and I told her I needed to go to the bank. She saw the briefcase in my hand and the look of despair on my face. She pleaded with me, "Garrett, please stay here. I really think it would be a good idea if you went to see Dr. Edwards. You've been acting really different that last couple of days. It's ok – I'll go with you." I became irritated instantly. "Hannah, stop. Every time I feel good about myself, you always try to bring me down. You have no idea what I've been up to the last few days!" She tried speaking to me as calm as possible. "I really think you're starting to become manic and you need medication." I lost it. I shouted, "I don't need medication and I don't have bipolar! You and my family are the crazy ones!" I turned around and left the apartment. I slammed the door behind me. My mind was racing. It was happening again. Everyone I loved was trying to stop me. I called a cab to a business down the street and walked down to wait.

The cab showed up and I jumped in. I told the driver I needed to go to Scotiabank. I was really chatty on the way there. I asked the cab driver if he had a business card, but he said he didn't like to give it out because Halifax was busy enough to pick up calls as they come. I asked him, "How would you like to stop driving a cab and drive a limousine for me someday soon?" He perked up instantly. "What kind of business are you running?" he asked. I told him I couldn't really discuss it at that time but that it would be huge. He quickly handed me his card and told me he would love to drive a limousine. I told him that his only responsibility would be to take me to and from meetings with different businesses around the city. We pulled up to the bank and as I got out of the car, he yelled, "Good luck in there!"

I walked into the bank and went right to the receptionist. I told her I needed a safety deposit box. She was very receptive and told me to follow her to the back room. I was impressed by the seemingly secure room. My concern laid in the fact that none of the spaces seemed large enough to fit my plastic tote. I expressed to the receptionist I needed something that could fit a three-foot by one-foot object. She said that she can make a few calls to companies that worked with the bank. I offered to look up some as well. She led me to a private room and I looked up companies. I stopped looking pretty quickly as my stress level was rising. I pictured Hannah calling my family and getting the cops after me again. I grabbed my phone and played rap music on maximum volume. I became fascinated by the messages the artists were sending me.

After a song or two, I heard a loud knock on the door. I stood up and opened it. A man in a suit was standing in front of me. I read his name tag. He was the branch manager. He told me I can't be playing my music at that volume as the whole bank could hear it. He asked me to sit with the receptionist to finish my business. I became more stressed and intensely irritable. "Whatever," I said to the manager. I sat down with the receptionist and asked her if she found anything yet. She was making phone calls but had had no luck yet. "Can you hurry up please, I'm kind of in a rush," I asked. She wasn't impressed with my tone. She replied, "I really don't like the way you're speaking to me; I think I've been very kind to you. Please have patience." I snapped back, "Oh, have patience? Listen to me! You have no idea what I've been through, ok? Don't tell me to have patience!" My leg was shaking with agitation. My eyes were wide open. I was fuming. She calmed down and asked me if I was okay.

She had a concerned look on her face. I stood up and yelled, "Everyone keeps asking me if I'm okay! No one will fucking do what I ask, though. You can't even find me a fucking box!" "I'm calling the police," she said. She quickly grabbed the phone and dialed 911. I continued screaming, "Good! Call the police! While you're at it, why don't you call the military police too? Tell them Lieutenant Garrett Campbell needs a ride!" She told me to please leave the bank. Everyone was staring at me. I told her to fuck off and stormed out.

Just as I was walking out the door, I could see Hannah's friend, Martha walking across the street on her way to the bank. "Oh, great! Here we go! You're here because Hannah was too scared to come herself! Is that right?" She was very calm when she spoke, "Garrett, it's ok. I'm here to help you. Hannah told me what happened earlier and she really wants you to get help." "Well don't worry, Martha! Help is on the way!" I replied. I sat down on the front steps of the bank and waited for the cops to show up. It only took a moment. It was the military police that arrived. They pulled onto the side of the road and I got up and walked over to them. They got out of the car and asked me to put the briefcase on the ground. I complied with their instructions. They asked me to open the briefcase. I popped it open and turned in towards them. They finally approached and looked inside only to find clothing and my passport. It wasn't what they were expecting. They kind of lightened up after seeing its contents. They were very polite but told me they would have to put cuffs on me for everyone's protection. I turned around and put my hands behind my back. He slapped on the cuffs.

They slowly walked me over to the car and put me in the back seat. They both got in and got on the radio talking about how they found me. The police had already been notified about me before my incident at the bank. I could only assume that Hannah had made some phone calls. I felt betrayed because I still didn't think there was anything wrong with me. I still thought I was missing a meeting with Facebook. All I had to do was keep my cool and find a place to store my tote. I knew that I messed up.

I asked the police if they could take me to the military base to see my doctor, but they pointed out that it was just after 4:00 pm so the base was closing. They got back on the radio, letting their team know that they were taking me to the hospital to be evaluated. My heart sunk. I really didn't want to be hospitalized again. Last time I had spent 30 days in the unit. I wasn't ready to do that again. I was also scared that I would miss my chance to meet with Facebook and discuss my plans.

During our drive, someone on the radio came through and asked the driver if he had confirmed the contents of the briefcase. He told the person on the other end there was just some clothing in it. I would later find out that the bank had told the police it was full of cash. I'm not sure where that idea came from, but it definitely didn't help the situation. We pulled up to the hospital about ten minutes after leaving the bank. They took me out of the car and told me they would take off the cuffs if I was going to continue to cooperate. I gave them my word and the cuffs came off. I walked into the hospital with one cop in front of me and the other behind me.

When I walked into the emergency room, all eyes were on me. Everyone was curious about why I was being escorted by police. I sat down to talk to the triage nurse. She put a device on my finger and asked me what was going on. One of the cops chimed in and told her they brought me here because I have bipolar disorder and they think I'm unwell. She asked a couple of follow-up questions and then they brought me to a private waiting room. I became very irritable over the next little while as I sat there with nothing to occupy my mind. It took about 30 to 40 minutes for someone to come in and see me, but it felt like 3 to 4 hours. I could barely sit still. I would go back and forth from sitting down and pacing around the room. I could feel another 30-day hospital stay approaching. I had to think of a way to get out. I remembered that I had paid Markus a retainer to help me out as my lawyer. Maybe he could get me out.

Eventually, a nurse came into the room. She sat down in front of me and asked me a question. The moment she finished, I looked at her right in the eyes and said, "Lawyer!" She explained to me that she was only there to help and she just needed some information from me to assess what's going on. "Lawyer!" I said once again. She continued to try and speak to me but each time she finished a sentence I would just scream "lawyer" at her. She eventually gave up and left the room. I fully expected the next person to walk in to have a phone with Markus on the line. I assumed I'd be let go in a matter of hours.

After 30 minutes, three staff members came into the room and asked me to follow them. They brought me down a hallway and told me to take a seat in a different room. There was a door in this room that led to a room of similar size. The door had a window on it, so I took a peek through the glass. I could see a woman in the other room standing in the middle of the room looking up and the ceiling speaking to someone. There was no one else in the room. I was confused as to who she was speaking with. Maybe she was like me. Maybe she had special powers, but they were different than mine. I tried to open the door to speak with her, but it was locked. I turned around and took a seat. A nurse came into the room shortly after and told me that Hannah was here and wanted to come to see me. I told her I wasn't ready to see her. I wanted Hannah to know that I was pissed off that she called the police about my situation. I would let her see me eventually, but I needed to send a message.

After a little while of waiting, I could see someone enter the room with the woman in it and bring her out. A nurse then came into my room to move me into the next room. When I got inside, I scanned around the room. I could see there were three doors. One to the room I was just in, one to the hallway, and one with no window. I didn't know where that door led to. I looked out the window into the hallway and I could see a bright orange sign partially blocking the hall. It read, "Staff Only." I quickly realized what was going on. The hospital was a base where they screen recruits to join the Earth's protection staff. I couldn't believe it. All this time, it's been right under my nose. The base was right in the middle of the city this whole time. Once you're screened in and designated as staff, you can visit the other side of the orange sign and see what's really going on. I needed to figure out how to prove to them I was ready to join them. I knew they were already interested based on what I had accomplished over the past few days.

I continued to investigate the room. I could see an emergency switch on the wall and two security cameras on the ceiling. They were watching me. I walked over to the emergency switch and analyzed it. It looked fake to me. I put one hand on the switch and stared into the camera. I flipped the switch down. Nothing happened. I was right, it was fake. I figured I had passed the test and could now proceed onto the next phase of the interview. I approached the third door without a window and tried to open it. Nothing. It was still locked. There must be something else that I was missing. I stood on the chair and pushed up the ceiling tiles looking for whatever I could find. I couldn't seem to figure out this puzzle.

Someone came into the room and told me to leave the ceiling tiles alone. I took that as advice that what I was looking for wasn't in the ceiling. I looked under the bottom side of the chair. Nothing. I was so confused. I wanted to join the staff so badly, but I couldn't figure out what I was supposed to do. While I was looking around the room frantically, I turned to the door and Hannah was standing there. I swallowed my pride and approached her. I gave her a long hug. I was happy to see her even though she betrayed me. I didn't feel comfortable telling her what was going on. She wouldn't understand that we were actually in one of Earth's recruitment centers. We sat on the bench together for what seemed like an eternity. After an hour, I couldn't take it anymore. I had to get out of there and figure out what the hell was going on. I stood up and opened the door to the hallway. I walked out into the hall and looked at the "Staff Only" sign. I wanted to walk past it, but I was nervous at first. I knew I wasn't done with my recruitment and it would be breaking the rules to move down that hallway. I looked at Hannah. I told her I wanted to join the staff. "What staff are you talking about, Garrett?" she asked. I raised my voice, "You wouldn't understand if I told you!" I turned away from Hannah and looked down the hallway. I took one step forward and screamed at the top of my lungs, "I WANT TO JOIN THE STAFF!"

I walked forward past the sign, I was now in their territory. Other powerful beings surrounded me. They asked me to go back to my room and take a seat. I looked at them and screamed, "I WANT TO JOIN THE FUCKING STAFF!" Security came from behind me and grabbed me. I didn't resist. After a moment, a woman approached and said, "You need to come with me." I agreed and the security let me go. I followed the woman back past the sign and into a dimly lit room. She pointed to a medical tablet and told me to lay down. The moment I got into position, security came into the room and tied my hands and feet down to the table. I felt uncomfortable with the situation. I squirmed, kicking my legs and trying to break free with my arms. Another woman entered the room with a needle. She walked over and stuck it into my shoulder. I was sure they were putting a chip in me. I could remember the conversation I had with my roommate during my first hospitalization. He told me they would put a chip in me eventually.

I looked around the room. I saw another fake-looking emergency switch on the wall. I thought to myself that all of this would end if I could just flip that switch. I tried to manipulate my body to free my arms. Nothing was working. I tried to move the entire table over to the wall. It was bolted to the floor. I started to aggressively jolt my body back and forth, trying to break free. I was getting unbelievably stressed. I screamed at the staff in the room with me. I was ordering them to free me, but no one would help. One woman told me they administered a medication and it should take effect soon. I yelled back, "Your medication won't do anything to me!" I knew that no matter what they gave me, I wouldn't be doing any sleeping. I was too wound up and I felt this way before. It's impossible to sleep when I feel this way. Security tried to hold me down and prevent me from flailing around. They couldn't stop me. I was twice as big as them and too strong.

The staff waited and waited for me to fall asleep, but I just kept throwing my body around and screaming at them. Eventually, the woman with the needle entered the room again with another dose. She approached the tablet and said, "We're doubling the dose." She looked at me and told me everything was going to be alright. She administered the dose. There was about another ten minutes of me flailing around before I started to doze off. Every time I started to dose off, though, I would fight with everything I had to stay awake. I didn't want to pass out; I wanted to leave the hospital. I fought it for as long as I could, but they untied me when they could tell I could barely move. They moved me off of the table and into a wheelchair. I was wheeled out of the room and down the hallway. We made a couple of turns and eventually arrived at an elevator. I assumed they were taking me to the basement to run experiments on me. They pushed me into the elevator and as it moved, I blacked out.

I woke up on a small mattress on the floor in the middle of an empty room. I felt like I had been hit by a bus. My mouth was dry like sandpaper. It was hard to open my eyes. I felt weak all over. As I made a failed attempt at standing up, a male nurse entered the room and helped me to my feet. He told me where I was. I was in unit 7A of the Halifax Infirmary; it was the psychiatric unit. I quickly asked the nurse if I could have some water. We made our way down the hall and stopped at the nursing station. He grabbed a cup of water and handed it to me. I chugged it. We continued down the hall and made our way into a three-person room. He showed me to my bed and I collapsed onto it. I wasn't ready to be up walking around. I needed more sleep. The medication was still keeping me down.

I fell back to sleep and woke up a little while later. I got up and went to the nurse's station to get more water, then headed back to my room. I looked around at my room. I thought that everything was a test. I didn't believe that I was in a real hospital. I was still manic and considered my situation as a form of basic training. I was being tested to see if I was ready to join Earth's staff. I quickly made all of the beds in the room and organized each area so that all three were the same. I standardized them. At basic training, you always had to keep a clean room, so I brought that knowledge here. I wanted to make sure I impressed whoever was watching me.

Eventually, two of my roommates entered the room. I knew right away that they weren't actual patients. I was sure that they were actors only here to watch me and report anything important back to their superiors. They questioned why I was touching their beds and I just ignored them. I would not take part in their games. I left the room and entered the hallway. There were more actors. They were all dressed as patients. I knew I had to be very careful with how I was acting. There were people watching me everywhere.

I stuck to myself for most of the day and eventually, a nurse came to find me. They said that they had some olanzapine for me. I knew I had to take it. I would never get to be part of Earth's staff if I didn't follow their rules. I took the medication and felt pretty tired a little while later. I made my way to my bedroom and laid down. I fell asleep quickly. As I was falling asleep, I could feel the actors in my room watching me and taking notes. I must have been so interesting to them – A regular human who knew all of their secrets.

The next day I woke up and was told I was going to meet with the doctor. I got myself ready and went to the appointment. While I was speaking with her, I started to second guess she was an actor. She kept asking me questions about bipolar disorder. I was feeling like I did during my first hospitalization. I felt trapped. I was expecting to finally get a briefing on what was next in the process of joining the staff, but she only wanted to discuss my illness. She was talking about her plan for medication while I was in hospital and what I would use at home. She told me I would be starting lithium as it was the gold standard for bipolar disorder. She also informed me she would keep the olanzapine going for a few weeks to make sure that we reverse the mania I'm experiencing.

My heart raced. Here I am trying to join the staff to protect Earth and she's labelling me as crazy. I became very agitated. Right after the appointment, I walked up to the nurse's station. I told them I wanted to leave immediately. They ignored me at first, so I raised my voice, "I'm a lieutenant in the Canadian Armed Forces and I demand that you let me go!" One nurse told me I have to lower my voice and that it's up to the physician when I go home. I tried one more time. "Let me go right now or I'm going to kick the fucking door down," I explained. They wouldn't budge. I stormed over to the security doors, stepped back from it and lunged at it with a powerful front kick. The door flew open. I could hear one of the nurses say, "Oh shit!" They didn't realize that I had superhuman strength.

I walked out the door and down the stairs slowly. I knew they would send people after me, so there was no point in running. I really just wanted to make a statement. When I got down two flights of stairs, five security guards came running down after me. When they got to me, I told them I would not resist or fight them. They asked me to walk back up the stairs, so I did. The nurses were huddled around the door I had kicked open when I got back to the unit. They led me to the solitary room and closed the door behind me as I entered. It was the room I had originally woke up in the day before. There was just a mattress on the ground and two security cameras on the ceiling. I didn't want them watching me anymore. I asked the nurse on the other side of the door for two cups of water. When I got them, I stared into the camera while I chugged them back. I then licked around the inside of the rim of the cup and stuck the cups to the cameras. They couldn't see me anymore.

A nurse came to the door quickly and told me I had to take the cups down. I responded by telling her I didn't want to be in there and that I would take them down if they let me back out. I explained to her I could have ran when I kicked the door open, but I didn't. I only kicked the door open because I said I would and I was ignored. She tried to make me a deal. She told me to take the cups down and if I'm well behaved for twenty minutes, she would let me out. I wanted out immediately but figured it would be the best deal I'd get. I took the cups down and laid on the mattress in the middle of the room flat on my back. I tried to sleep, but I was too wired. I just laid there with my eyes closed. Eventually, the twenty minutes passed and I was let out. I had learned my lesson that I had to play by the rules or I'd be stuck in that room alone and bored to death.

I stayed on my best behavior from that moment moving forward. I just wanted to get out of the hospital as fast as possible. With each passing day, I would think less and less about the Earth's staff and how everyone was an actor. The olanzapine was resetting my mind out of the mania and back to normal. The nurses gave me passes to go to the gym and participate in yoga classes. We had painting classes, group meditation, and they even let me play some basketball here and there. Staff from work came to visit me once and Hannah was in daily after the first couple of days had passed. Like the first episode, I was hospitalized for just over 30 days before being released.

When I got home from the hospital, I looked around the apartment. I had remembered doing certain things that were pretty out of the ordinary. I saw my briefcase in the computer room and had a flashback of buying it at staples and taking it with me on my meeting with Evan. I opened the closet door and saw my computer thrown in next to a tote covered in garbage bags. I remembered packing it all up and taking my computer apart. I walked out onto the balcony and saw butts on the ground from the joints I had been smoking. I remember thinking to myself, "What the hell is wrong with me?" I made a promise to myself at that moment I would take the lithium for the rest of my life. I didn't want anything like this happening again. It's just too bad that the lithium wouldn't be enough and my mania wasn't done with me.

EPISODE 3

MY HOSPITAL RELEASE WAS ON A FRIDAY, SO I HAD THE WEEKEND to get my life reorganized. On the first day, I cleaned up the butts from the joints, set my computer back up, and unpacked the tote full of books and objects from around the room. It was hard to look at the tote. I couldn't understand why I was thinking the way I was thinking. Why did I think a survey on Facebook was an application? Why did I think that they were sending people to pick me up? Why did I think commercials were designed for me as a set of special instructions? I found all of this hard to deal with.

I spent a lot of time over the next few months discussing my issues with my psychologist. We tried to work through my deep-seeded depression and came to the consensus I never really got over my childhood. I never got past watching my mother pass away and living with an alcoholic as a father. I was too young when everything fell apart and didn't have a normal upbringing since the age of ten. All of the nights of finding my father drunk and passed out stuck with me. The numerous times I had to help him get to bed while he cried for his wife to come back were still in my mind. I still thought of the night he almost killed me while he was drinking and driving. I reached out onto the road to wave to him and he swerved towards me. I was barely able to jump out of the way. I had a perfect life until my mother was diagnosed with cancer. After that, everything was just really tough.

I worked with her twice a week for months trying to put things into perspective. She tried to get me to focus on the great parts of my family I do have. I have a wonderful brother and sister plus lots of first cousins that I'm close with. She also wanted me to change the story in my mind. Instead of looking at myself at a victim, she wanted me to look at my situation as something that I have overcome. Despite losing my mother and having a rough home life, I still got myself into pharmacy school and succeed in it. She talked about how difficult it was to achieve this. I played along with her, but none of this was really working for me. In my mind, my childhood would always be something I look at negatively. I just assumed she didn't understand how hard it really was. I didn't care about overcoming it. I just wished that I didn't have to go through it. There would never be a moment where I didn't miss my mother, and I would never forgive my father for not being there for me. It was pretty simple in my mind. I would always be depressed, but I would just have to make things work and live my life. My main concern was to not become manic again so I could stop spending money and get my student loan paid off.

Life finally stabilized until Hannah finished school that year and graduated from pharmacy at Dalhousie. After she got her exam marks back, she worked in Amherst, which was a couple of hours away. This meant I was alone in Halifax. I became really sad when she left, and it slowly turned into a bout of depression. I was getting no comfort from going to work because it was just a constant reminder I would be released from the military, which made me feel like I wasn't good enough. I was playing basketball with the base team and I really found that it did help, but eventually word came down from the higher-ups I would not be able to compete at regionals or nationals because of my medical category, so I quit playing. It seemed like everything in my life was falling apart. I couldn't play basketball anymore; my girlfriend was away from me and I was still waiting for my military career to end.

The depression set in hard. I made it to work for the first couple weeks, but I was a mess before and after. Most days when I got home from work, I would leave my uniform on and get right into bed at 4:00 pm. I would stay in bed until my hunger forced me to get up and feed myself. I would usually choose something easy like a bowl of cereal. Eventually, I ran out of food and had to go get a grocery order. I can remember the anxiety I had in my chest with the thought of being out in public. I sweated from my forehead and could feel my heart pounding. I felt like everyone who saw me would think there was something wrong with me or that I was acting strange. I also had a never-ending fear of having another manic episode. I got in my car and drove to the grocery store, but when I parked in the parking lot, I couldn't get myself to get out of the car. I was watching all of the people go in and out of the store, and I was scared to join them. I had to call Hannah to get a pep talk and have her tell me I could do it. She eventually told me to get out of the car and walk into the store. I was nearly having a panic attack. I made her stay on the phone with me the entire time. She would pick an item and tell me to find it. I couldn't even think straight about what I needed to make meals, so I just listened to what she told me. She would say things like, "Ok, Garrett, now look for bananas. Tell me when you see them. Alright now grab some and put them in your cart. Now look for apples." I followed her instructions and got through it. I tried to get as many things as possible that didn't require preparation. I wanted things I could just grab and eat. When it was time to check out, I was too nervous to stand in line with other people, so I took the time to go to the self-checkout. I eventually made it out of the store and back to my car. I sat in the driver seat, taking deep breaths. It was a tough experience for me to have so much anxiety and go to a public place. I really didn't want to have to do that alone again. Hannah stayed on the phone with me for a few more minutes before I had to drive home.

The depression only got worse as time went on. I eventually started calling in sick to work and stayed in bed all day. I got to where I wasn't eating. I recall one day I was caught in the same cycle as my first bout of depression where I was too hungry to sleep but too tired to get up and make myself food. I gagged in bed with hunger, but I couldn't get myself to the kitchen. I knew I had to do something, but I could do nothing on my own. I wanted to get Hannah on the phone, but she was at work so I sucked it up and called my sister. I was extremely embarrassed when she answered. Here I was, a grown adult military pharmacy officer lying in bed gagging because I couldn't make myself a snack. She said hello and I instantly told her, "I'm really not doing good, Mel."

Whenever my sister hears something like that she instantly springs into action. She asked me what exactly was going on and I told her that I'm going through another depressed phase and that I was scared. I was honest with her and told her that I was gagging in bed due to hunger and was thinking about killing myself again. I just couldn't take the embarrassment of what happened during my last episode and I felt like I was worthless because the military was releasing me.

She coached me. She told me to sit up on the bed and put my feet on the floor. I listened to her instructions. She then broke down the plan for me. "Alright, Garrett, here's what's going to happen. You're going to get up and go into the kitchen. You'll open the fridge and find anything you can to make a sandwich. I'll walk you through it every step of the way, but you have to listen to me and just get to the fridge. After you eat your sandwich, you're going to call the base and make an appointment with your psychiatrist. Does that sound like a good plan to you?" I really didn't want to go to the base, but I knew Melissa was looking out for my best interest. I agreed that it would work.

"Ok, Garrett, stand up," she instructed me. I could feel a sharp pain in my stomach when I stood up straight. I was more comfortable to be hunched over. She continued, "Walk out of the bedroom and get to the kitchen. It's ok, I'm right here." I walked out slowly gagging again with hunger. "Open the fridge and grab mayonnaise, sandwich meat, and cheese." I found all of the items. "Open the bread and take out two pieces. Open the mayo and put some on each piece of bread. Do you have a knife? Get a knife." I grabbed the knife and put mayo on the bread. "You're almost there, Garrett. Cut a few pieces of cheese and open the sandwich meat." My stomach growled with the anticipation of the food to come. I had never been so empty. "Put the cheese and meat onto the bread and put in together. Take a bite as soon as you can." My stomach let out another massive growl as I took my first bit. It tasted so good. I felt like I hadn't eaten in days. I devoured the sandwich. I put Melissa on speakerphone so I could eat it with two hands. It was hard to stop and give myself time to chew. When I finished eating it, Ashely told me I needed to get a drink of water and that we will make another sandwich. She talked me through the process again, and I eventually made and ate a second one. She instructed me to go sit on the couch and get ready to call the base. After talking for a little while longer, she said it was time to call them and that she would call me back in a little while to check in. She stressed how important it was to get in with my psychiatrist.

We hung up the call and called the base to make my appointment. It was scheduled for two days' time. I was anxious about going, but I knew that it was the right move since I was thinking about killing myself again. I just wanted something to help stop the constant thoughts of self-harm. Now that the appointment was made and I had food in my stomach, I made my way back to bed. This time, I was able to fall asleep. The next morning, I checked the mail. It was the most productive thing I had done in days. There was a piece of mail from Scotiabank inside. When I opened it, I found a letter explaining that due to my behavior at the bank in prior months, they could no longer serve me. This was just more negativity to add to my spiraling mind.

Two days later, I went to my appointment and we got me started back on sertraline to help get me out of the depressed phase of bipolar disorder I was experiencing. They reassured me that things would get better, but I didn't see how it was possible this time. Would I magically stop focusing on the fact that I'm getting released from the military? Would I stop caring I was getting paid $20,000 less than my peers because I have a mental illness? Would I stop missing my basketball team and the sport itself? These issues seemed real and they didn't seem like they were going anywhere. I felt like I was stuck.

Things did eventually get better, though. As the months went by, I eventually made it back to work full time and focused on the positives. Since I was getting medically released, it meant that I wouldn't have to get posted to another part of Canada and be away from Hannah. This would eventually give us the opportunity to move back to Sydney, where I grew up and be close to my family and my cottage. Hannah left her position in Amherst and found a job in Halifax, so we were back together again. This made a big difference for me. It meant a lot to have her back in my day to day life. Another positive thing that happened was that a position opened up at the base pharmacy for a full-time civilian pharmacist. Everyone that I worked with told me I should apply for it. I was hesitant at first just because my boss knew I had bipolar disorder so I assumed that they wouldn't hire me back on, but I went forward with the application because it was a huge opportunity and I knew that Hannah wanted to stay in Halifax for a bit longer before we moved home.

I handed in my resume to the contracting company and later had my interview. The position was granted so I wrote a memo to change my medical release date to a month earlier. Everything was approved, and before I knew it, I was a civilian working at the base. It was strange for me to be working there and no longer be in the military, but I was so happy to be making a pharmacist salary for the first time in my life. It felt like I was finally being treated fairly. Everything seemed to go well enough to stop taking my sertraline for depression. My psychiatrist was hesitant to keep me on it when things were going good due to the risk of it pushing me into mania. I stayed on my lithium and kept the attitude I would be on it forever. Lithium was my mood stabilizer, so it was important to keep it on board.

Things went well at work for the following 8 months. I was giving pain presentations to military members suffering from chronic pain. I was taking part in an addictions day program where I would give presentations to members struggling with addiction. I worked in the pharmacy checking prescriptions and counselling patients on new medications. I was totally in the zone and was loving my job there. I felt like everything worked out for the best.

During the eighth month, however, my optimism grew to a concerning level. It all started one day after work when I had the idea to start a YouTube channel where I would discuss medications. I always wanted to have a YouTube channel but never knew what sort of topics I would cover. I checked out a couple of medications in YouTube search and noticed there weren't too many drug channels out there. I created a channel and called it Drug Talk. For three days in a row, I would make a video once I got home from work. After the third day, I had grandiose thoughts about my channel and thought that one day, I would have the biggest drug channel on YouTube. I imagined having 1,000,000 subscribers and generating a side revenue stream with the channel to match my income. Once the grandiose ideas started, my sudden craving for cannabis came back. I knew deep down that cannabis was a bad idea for me, but something inside of me kept me craving it and eventually, I crumbled to my desire.

This time, instead of contacting a dealer, I went to a cannabis clinic operating seemingly illegally. I didn't understand how they sold cannabis to anyone with a driver's license, but it was very convenient, nonetheless. I bought a couple of different brands and went back to my apartment. It was a Friday night. Hannah was working 10 pm to 8 am so I had all night to do whatever I wanted. I got back to the apartment and rolled a joint. I took it up to the park and smoked it. Once I finished it, I felt a heightened sense of self-worth. I felt like I was amazing for thinking of the idea for the YouTube channel and I couldn't wait to make it big. I had finally found something that didn't cost any money but could generate an income. It was my replacement for Arbonne from years past.

I went back to the apartment and watched videos about how to grow a YouTube channel from scratch. I watched videos for hours and every hour I would go out and smoke another joint. Each time I came back inside, my thoughts would be more grandiose. After my third joint, I looked up conspiracy theory videos and eventually landed on illuminati videos. While I was watching them, I took everything as the truth. In one video they talked about selling your soul to join the illuminati and signaling to the world by doing one eye symbolism. I knew what I had to do. If I wanted my YouTube channel to get big, I would have to sell my soul by posting a picture of myself doing one eye symbolism. I ran to my closet and put on a blue dress shirt. I grabbed a bottle of Tylenol and took it to the living room. I took out a Tylenol and held it between my index finger and thumb and stuck my pinky finger, ring finger, and middle finger straight up. I was making the 666 symbol from the illuminati videos I had watched. I looked through the hole I was making with one eye and took a selfie. I instantly posted it as my Facebook profile picture. Now everyone would know. I was the illuminati's pharmacist. I would educate the world on medication for them and in return, they would grant me riches.

I was very excited that I had figured this out. I went outside to smoke another joint to celebrate. While I was smoking it, the truth from my last manic episode came back. I remembered the truth about my reality. I couldn't believe that I had forgotten. I was still in the matrix this whole time. How did I forget? I went months without thinking about it while I could have been taking advantage of my situation. Not everyone was lucky like me to know the truth about reality. I went out into the matrix to take a look at what I've been missing out on.

I took the elevator down to the parking garage and hoped into my Ford Escape. I went to Wendy's to get some food. While I was driving around, I remember looking around in awe. The matrix was so beautiful. All the streetlights seemed like they were different colors than before. Once you realize what reality is, it must change. I looked at the people on the sidewalk as I passed them. I felt bad they didn't know what was going on. They seemed to do all right though. I couldn't waste time feeling bad for others. I had too much important stuff to handle. I eventually got to Wendy's and ordered some food in the drive through. I parked in the parking lot to eat. I was observing every fry. I thought to myself, "Man, the matrix really does have some good food." I felt so lucky to be realizing everything. While I was eating the burger, I was questioning if it's even real. It was delicious but was it really in my hands? Was I tasting it or was the matrix just putting thoughts of taste into my mind? I would have to do more thinking about that later. For now, I just wanted to enjoy the experience.

After I finished eating, I started slowly driving home. About halfway there, I was approaching a BMW dealership. The sign was lit up by a white light and I took that as a sign I was supposed to go into the parking lot and look at what they offered. I realized quickly that I could have whatever car I wanted. Whatever you thought of in the matrix could easily transpire. I slowly drove between the lines of cars until one caught my eye. It was a navy blue 2013 328xi. It was listed for $27,000. I thought about how much money I will be making as the illuminati's pharmacist. This was nothing for me to afford. I would eventually make more than that every month. I got out of my Escape and looked closely. It was what I always wanted. It had beige interior with wood finishes. It was a beautiful car. I decided at that moment I would return the next day to pick it up.

I got back into my car feeling excited. I couldn't believe that I would finally have a BMW of my own. I sped back home and rolled up a joint to celebrate. I would usually take it to the park, but I didn't care about the no smoking rules. I was untouchable. I brought it out onto the patio to smoke it. When I came back in, I turned on the TV to see what messages there were for me. I flipped through the channels until I noticed a scene of a show with vampires. I paused on it. I couldn't believe what I was watching. Why was the matrix trying to tell me about vampires? It could only mean one thing; they were coming for me. Vampires were real in the matrix.

I had to think fast. I was instantly concerned about Hannah's safety. Were they coming for me and Hannah was here, she would be in danger. I ran to the kitchen and opened up the cupboards. I was looking for a spray bottle that Hannah used to water our plants. I finally found it and filled it up with water. I opened the fridge and found a couple of cloves of garlic. I grated them up with a cheese grater and placed the pieces into the spray bottle. I ran down the hall towards the door of the apartment shaking the spray bottle as I ran. I got to the door and sprayed it along the edges. I put a good coat on it. After I sprayed it for about 5 minutes, I felt like I was safe. I hid the bottle next to my computer and took a seat. I was still scared, but I knew I did everything right. I kind of felt like a genius. There was no way they were getting in.

I spent the rest of the night watching videos on how to grow a YouTube channel. I wanted to learn everything I could about how to make it successful. I knew that it wasn't necessary, though. I had sold my soul to the illuminati so it was just a matter of posting videos and letting them handle the rest. But I still wanted to prove that I would work for my success. I watched videos for hours periodically checking the stats on my channel. I had about 50 subscribers. I could feel it that that number would explode someday.

I eventually got in bed and continued to watch videos on my phones. I stayed awake until Hannah got home from work the next morning and I got up to share some exciting news with her. "Hey, babe. Listen. I want to tell you something, but I really don't want you to be scared or have any concerns. I'm buying a BMW today!" I was hyped up while I told her. She replied, "Garrett, you always talk about how stupid it is to buy expensive cars. I don't understand why the sudden change of heart. I really think you should talk to your doctor as soon as possible. I've been concerned about you for a couple of days now." I became irate. "You always try to bring me down once I start feeling good about myself! I've been through a lot and I want to buy something nice! It's not that big of a deal! I make more than enough money to get it!" She pleaded, "Garrett please don't do this. You're going to regret it."

I was done with the conversation. How could she find a way to not support me when she supposedly loves me so much? I went into the bedroom and got dressed. "What're you doing, Garrett? Are you going somewhere?" She asked me. I decided to lie and told her I would get something to eat. I left the apartment, got in my car and drove to the BMW dealership.

I walked in and approached what I thought was the receptionist. I told her that there's a car in the lot that I'd like to test drive. She brought me outside, and I showed her the car from the night before. She went inside to grab the keys and we got inside. She drove at first to show off some features. Eventually we pulled into a parking lot and switched so I could drive. I drove around Halifax for 20 minutes. I liked the way it drove. It was something that I wanted to have. It felt so much better than my Ford Escape. I asked her if there was a place we could go so I could test sports mode. She gave me directions until we got to an old side road down by some railroad tracks. I lined the car up in the road and turned on sports mode. I paused for a moment. It was silent in the car. She looked at me and said, "You're not going to do anything crazy are you?" I laughed and told her I would behave. I put the pedal down to the floor and took off. I could see the speedometer soaring up past 60, 80 and then to 100. Once it passed 100 km/hr I put on the break and slowed the car down. I looked at her and said, "I'll take it."

We drove back to the dealership and she said there was some paper-work I had to fill out. I filled everything out and then asked her if I could have the car today. She told me that unfortunately, I had to wait until the following day so they could prepare the car and contact Scotiabank for financing. My impulse was to tell her that I'm not financing it through Scotiabank after they cut me off as a client, but I didn't want to share the details with her so I let it slide. She told me to come back first thing tomorrow morning and they would have it ready for me. She also told me I had the option to trade in my escape. "Consider it done," I said.

I drove home a little disappointed that I wasn't driving my new car, but I tried to keep focused on what mattered. Hannah was safe from Vampires and I was in the illuminati. Everything was ok. I parked my car at home and walked over to the bakery nearby. I ordered the best breakfast and best desert they had and grabbed a latte with it. I sat down to eat and went back to thinking about how much I love being in the matrix. I loved how whatever I wanted was mine. I had only to show some initiative and ask for what I want. I thought about how many wonderful moments I would have in the coming years now that I knew the truth. I eventually found a way to share the truth with Hannah as well so we could live out our dreams together harnessing the power of the matrix.

After I finished eating, I made my way back to my apartment. I was quiet when I went inside as I knew Hannah would be asleep. She slept all day when she was on her work week. I went into the living room to get more information from the television. During the first commercial break, a Telus ad appeared advertising a new deal for the Samsung Galaxy 9S+. I was amazed; the matrix was even telling me which phone I needed to buy. I shut off the television and got ready to head to the mall. I snuck out the garlic covered door and got into my car. I exited the parking garage and drove to the Halifax Shopping Center. When I walked in, I was amazed at how much I could get there. Anything I wanted was mine. There were so many stores to visit. I had to stay on task, though. I was ordered to get a Samsung Galaxy, so I had to get to Telus.

I eventually came across the store and walked in. They asked me what they could help me with and I told them I saw an ad on the television for the Galaxy S9+ and I'd like to get one. I sat down with one employee and he brought up my file. He asked me if I would be trading in my iPhone and I told him I would be. He then listed off some promotional offers. He told me I could get the special headphones for the phone at a discount price. I told him to throw them in. He mentioned that the 3D camera was available and would work great with my phone. "I'll take it," I said. I looked over his shoulder and saw the virtual reality headset. He saw me looking at it and asked if it interested me. I told him to ring in one of those. He understood that I was willing to spend money and he showed me a SONOS speaker with Alexa built in. I would have bought anything he suggested. I told him to put it in the bag.

I didn't think of my situation as being at a Telus store. I was in a matrix hub I was ordered to visit through the television. I felt like I was buying the equipment needed to accomplish my goals in the matrix. Anything he offered me, I bought. I took his suggestions as orders. I needed to buy whatever he told me about. It wasn't a matter of choice but of necessity. I left the store that day with over $2000 worth of electronics.

I walked down the mall checking every store that caught my eye. After a couple of stores, I found myself in a jewelry store. They were having a special promotion with custom jewelry. A man was there to make customers unique items that weren't available in store. I knew this couldn't be a coincidence. I approached him and asked him if he could make something with emeralds. He told me he loves working with emeralds and asked me what I was looking for. I said that that was my birthstone and I was thinking maybe a ring would be nice. He showed me pictures of what he could do with diamonds and said that he could swap out the diamonds for emeralds if anything interests me. I loved everything I laid my eyes on. I finally picked out a ring that would have nine emeralds in it. He mentioned that he could make that for me for about $2500. I was sold. I told him to make it and gave him my name and number. I left the store with a massive smile on my face.

I wanted to keep shopping, but I knew I had to get home to set up my new electronics. I left the mall. While I drove home, I had my window down and I was moving my hand up and down through the wind. I was still puzzled with how real everything felt. I knew deep down it was all fake, but it was so hard to tell from the inside. I wanted to get to the core of the matrix someday and see what it was all for. I thought that maybe my virtual reality headset I just purchased would take me to a second level. Maybe it would reveal a second dimension to the system. The thought of this excited me.

I made it back to my apartment and opened the new electronics I purchased. I put in the ear bud headphones and blasted some rap. I felt like an agent from The Matrix movie when I had them in my ears. They were so sleek. Then it dawned on me - maybe I'm being trained to become a matrix agent. I had the military training and I knew the truth of reality. It made so much sense. I wanted to go into the matrix on foot with my new equipment. I rolled a joint and went outside to walk to the park.

While I was walking, I could see the odd person look at the buds in my ears. I felt like they were fearing me because they knew that I was a powerful agent in the making. They knew to stay away from me and leave me to my business. I didn't want anyone to get hurt, but I wouldn't hesitate to protect myself if I needed to. I got into the park and lit my joint. I stared up at the clouds while I puffed it. I had so many questions in my mind. I wanted to know my mission. What was my purpose? I knew that the only thing I could do was to follow the hints left and keep doing my best to receive communication from the controllers. I knew I would have my questions answered eventually.

After I finished smoking, I went back out near the street and sat on a bench. I was watching the people walk by wondering who knew what was going on and who was just letting the matrix control their lives.

I imagined a world where everyone was awake to the truth and we all worked together to figure this whole thing out. I felt like it was my duty to protect those who were still asleep. I knew it was the duty of a matrix agent and I didn't want to disappoint. I sat there for about 30 minutes and then headed back to my apartment. I spent the rest of the night smoking joints and looking forward to getting my new car in the morning.

When the next day rolled around, I got up at 8:00 am and put on the nicest clothing I could find in my closet. I wore a white button up shirt with a matching pair of grey dress pants and a blazer. I left without eating breakfast and went right to the dealership. I approached the woman that took me for the test drive and told her I was there to pick up my car. She had some paperwork ready for me. Some of it had to be filled out on the spot and some had to be taken to the DMV. They had a driver there that was ready to take me. I handed her the keys to my Escape for the trade in. It took about an hour to go to the DMV and register the vehicle then we drove back to the dealership. When we returned, I took pictures and posting them to social media. I wanted everyone to know that I was getting a BMW.

The woman helping me was going back and forth from my car to her office taking care of different tasks and I stopped her at one point and asked her if I could sit in the car for a moment. She gave me the keys and told me there is still some paperwork to fill out before the sale is complete, but it was fine to go look at it. I went outside and got into the car. I couldn't wait to leave and go for a joy ride. As I sat there, I recalled that I would be a matrix agent and would soon run the matrix. This meant that I can do whatever I want. If I said the car was mine, it was mine. Who were these people to tell me I had to fill out more forms? They didn't know what I knew. I had waited long enough. It was time for this car to be mine. I looked in the rear-view mirror and seen the woman come out of the building towards the car. I pressed the ignition and started the car. She walked a little faster toward me. I put the car in drive and slowly moved forward. I could see the woman run and got to the car. She was banging on the back of the car telling me to stop. I hit the gas and peeled off the lot. I could see her in the rear-view mirror waving her arms in the air screaming at me.

I didn't care about other people's rules. They were taking too long to the sell me the car so I made it mine. I took the car because they weren't moving along fast enough. I didn't have time to wait for their bullshit. I rolled down the windows and put my arm out to feel the air once again. I felt like I was a god driving around Halifax. Everyone who could see me knew I was on a different level. I could feel my abilities return from the summer of 2014.

Then I had a thought. I thought that because I was so powerful, the military would probably want to sit down and talk with me. They couldn't have an agent running around Halifax unless they knew I was on their team. I loved the military so the least I could do was to sit down with them and discuss my intentions here on Earth. I took a quick trip to the mall to replace my outfit. I pulled into the parking lot and walked into the mall. I looked at my phone and seen missed calls from Hannah and my friend, Noah. I didn't have time to call them back. I had more important stuff to take care of.

I went inside and walked right to Tip Top Tailor's. I walked up to the counter and told them I wanted to replace my outfit with sizes that fit better. I wanted the same outfit, just a new pair of pants and a new button up shirt. I took off my blazer and the worker measured me. He then gave me a few options to try on. I went into the dressing room to change. Everything fit perfectly. I knew it would because they knew I was coming in advance and had everything ready for me. Everyone knew who I was and would do anything to assist me in my mission. I put my old clothes in a bag, paid with credit card, and left feeling like a million bucks. I wanted to continue to shop, but I knew I had to get to the base. I left the mall and made my way to CFB Halifax.

As I approached the gate, I felt nervous. I knew this was a big moment for humanity. It would be the first time that a matrix agent met with the Canadian Forces. History would be made. I showed my ID at the gate and drove in. As I turned to my right, I noticed a police car sitting there. I found it weird because it wasn't military police. It was regional officers. They instantly turned their lights on and pulled up behind me. I pulled over and put my hands on the wheel. An officer got out of his car and approached my window. I rolled it down and he ask me, "Are you Garrett Campbell?" I acknowledged that I was. "You know that this car is stolen right? We were just talking with the BMW dealership and they said you pulled off the lot before the paperwork was finished." I played dumb. I responded, "I thought everything was cleared up, they already drove me to the DMV and we registered the car under my name." I doubt they bought it, but they played along. "Why don't you drive back to the dealership and have a talk with them. We're going to follow you back over." I agreed. I turned the car back on and did a U-turn. I felt bad for not making the meeting with the military staff. I knew how disappointed they would be.

I drove back to the dealership slowly. The police followed me the entire way. When I pulled into the parking lot, I could see Hannah standing there. I parked the car, got out and gave her a hug. Then I looked at her and said, "Don't try to stop me." I went inside and told them I was here to fill out the rest of the paper work. Hannah came in behind me and the police came in after. Hannah pleaded with the police not to let me buy this car. She told them I have Bipolar Disorder and that I don't actually want to buy it. She said that I need to be seen by a doctor. I looked back at the cops and told them that Hannah has no right to tell me what I can or cannot buy. I reminded them she was my girlfriend, not my wife. She has no control over my finances. The police told Hannah they have no power to stop me from buying a car if I wanted to. Hannah cried. She didn't understand why no one would listen to her. To this day, I still don't understand why they wouldn't stop me. I just stole a car right off the lot. Something was going on.

I went into the office with the salesperson and Hannah stayed out in the lobby with the police. I signed everywhere the man told me to sign. He told me the interest rate was 4.52% from Scotiabank and I initialed next to it. He asked me if I wanted rim protection for $1300. I said, "Of course." I signed for it and he added it to the price. I initialed a few more spots on the paperwork and then he stood, up shook my hand and said, "Congratulations, Garrett. The car is yours."

I left the office and walked out of the building hand in hand with Hannah. She was still shaken up, but I think she was ultimately happy that I was ok and didn't get arrested. I told her I was sorry I had to be so stern with her; I just didn't want her to stop me from getting the car. We drove back to our apartment and went inside. I gave Hannah another hug, told her I loved her, and apologized for scarring her. She told me I need to talk to my doctor. She was worried something would happen . I told her that I will work the next day so if anyone thinks anything is going on, I'll talk to Dr. Edwards.

The next day, I got up for work and got myself dressed. I was excited for my first day at work as a matrix agent. I knew I couldn't talk openly about it, but I would enjoy myself. I had figured that everyone in the pharmacy I worked with were all actors and they were just playing the role of colleagues. I assumed that they were there to watch over me and make sure that I had everything I needed to complete my work. When I got to work that day, I was overly enthusiastic. I had a great conversation with every patient that came to the counter. Around mid-morning, some high-ranking officers came to the pharmacy to pick up medication. I assumed picking up medication was a cover and that they were actually here to see me. I said little; I just gave them what they asked for. When they were leaving, one of them stared into my eyes and thanked me for the quick service. I took this as a sign. Maybe that was a signal. Maybe every person that made eye contact with me was similar to myself and was in some way aware of the matrix.

For the remainder of the morning, I tried to look every person in the eyes when I was talking to them. To my surprise, most kept eye contact. Was everyone in the military aware of reality as I saw it? Were they just sending people to see me that were aware? I was so intrigued. Right before lunch started, I had to take a patient into the side counselling room to check his blood pressure. While I was testing it, he kept talking about the new Halifax Central Library and how he was going there after he left the base. I took a mental note of this. After I was done with him it was lunch time. I put on my jacket and left the pharmacy, proceeding to the front doors of the building. Hannah was supposed to pick me up for a lunch date, but I didn't see her in the parking lot. I started walking back to our apartment to see what she was doing.

There were only three cars in the parking lot and one was facing the side walk. As I walked past it, I saw a girl roughly my age sitting behind the wheel. She looked up and locked eyes with me. I knew this was a signal. I walked up to the passenger side door and opened it. I looked at her and said, "Listen, I'm going to get in your car and if at any point you feel uncomfortable or want me to leave just say so and I'm gone." She didn't tell me to go. She was very inviting. I got in her car and she asked me where I needed to go. I told her to take me to the Halifax Central Library. She pulled out of the parking lot without any questions asked. I assumed she was expecting me to get in her car and that she already knew where I was going.

As we drove to the library we didn't talk too much. She tried to make a little small talk but I kind of shrugged off the conversation. I was too focused on discovering what was going on in my own mind. Why was everyone showing themselves now? Did they realize that I reached their level all on my own? We made it to the library and she pulled all the way around the building into a small parking lot on the far side of the building. I looked at her and she said, "You're on your own now, man." I assumed that that meant she was just a driver and wasn't privy to more information. I thanked her for the drive and got out of the car.

There were lots of people standing outside of the library. A few had Tim Horton's coffee cups. I took that as a sign they were people I was supposed to interact with. I walked up to one of them standing by himself. I said hello, but he said little back. I noticed a piece of paper hanging out of his pocket. Was it a note for me? I reach down to grab it, but the man told me not to touch him. I didn't want to waste any more time with him. I turned away from him and walked into the library. I saw people in the back on computers so I walked down. One of them looked at me and stared at me in the eyes for a moment. It was just what I needed. I sat down right next to him and tried to log on to the computer. He told me I needed a library card to get access and pointed to the receptionists. I got up from the computer and walked over to them and told them I'd like to sign up for a membership. They showed me a couple of different cards to choose from. One of them had a picture of an alien on it. I was intrigued. Was this another sign? Were aliens involved in this? I chose the alien photo card.

They got me signed up and I went back over to the computers. Someone had taken my seat, but I noticed a seat open next to someone with a Tim Horton's cup. I sat down next to them. After I logged in, I asked him how he was doing. He told me, "I'm doing fine. I'm just having trouble working on this project. I work for a large organization that is working towards removing sugar and other bad foods from the school system." I felt like I was being recruited. I talked to him about it for a little while and he gave me his number so I could attend a meeting sometime. I checked the clock and realized that I had about 40 minutes until I had to be back at work after lunch break. I checked out the rest of the library. I knew that I would be spending a lot of time in the coming months so it would be a good idea to get a lay of the land.

I walked up the stairs to the second floor. I noted what each section offered as I walked around the floor. After I was satisfied, I went up to the third floor. There were many people on computers there. A few had Tim Horton's cups so I walked behind them to see what messages they had up for me on their computer screens. One of them had a picture of a black hole. As soon as I looked at it, she switched the screen to an article about multiple dimensions. She was feeding me the exact information I needed. It made so much sense. I was entering into another dimension. How could I not have realized this sooner? The entire time I thought I was in the matrix, but in fact I had entered into another dimension with different people and different abilities. I hurried up to the fourth floor. When I arrived, I looked out the window and saw Tim Horton's down the street. I knew that that was where I needed to go. Everyone was signaling me to go there.

I took the elevator to the lobby and rushed out of the library. As soon as I walked outside, the sun shined for me. I looked around at all of the people who had moved into a higher dimension with me. It was beautiful. I could hear the birds chirping more clearly. The air felt crisp. Everything was perfect. I walked down the street towards Tim Horton's. I was trying to look everyone in the eyes as they passed me by. I thought back to my library card and quickly realized that in this dimension, there wasn't just humans. Extraterrestrials were walking the streets with me. They knew that I had finally realized that they were there and they enjoyed that fact that I knew who they were. I wondered what star system they came from. Was it a nearby star or somewhere else? Knowing they were multidimensional made me think that they were here all along.

While I was walking down the street, I passed by CIBC Bank. A young gentleman was inside and we locked eyes while I was passing by. I had to go in and talk to him. I opened the door and told him my name. I reached my hand out to shake his hand. He introduced himself and I asked him what sort of a business he was creating. I could tell by looking at him he was in some entertainment role. He told me he was trying to start a label. I was impressed. I told him that I'm a YouTuber and asked if he recommended CIBC. He said it was a great place and told me I should definitely move my accounts there. I felt like he was sending a direct message to me. I had to become a member of that bank. I grabbed some pamphlets and told him I had to go and it was nice to meet him. I was running out of time.

I made it to Tim Horton's and went inside to buy a coffee. I wanted to signal to others that I knew what was going on and that I was a part of the team. I decided at that moment that everyone with a red cup was a Canadian with the capacity to enter higher dimensions. While I was in line, I saw a Halifax newspaper laying on the ground. When I picked it up, it was opened to the horoscopes. I read Taurus's. I was blown away. It dictated my life perfectly. I never knew that horoscopes had so much meaning. I promised myself that I would never miss reading my horoscope again. They were direct messages from higher dimensional beings. It was everything I needed to know about my day. I thought commercials were the best way to get instructions, but horoscopes made way more sense. Everything was becoming bigger and bigger. The scope of reality was blowing my mind.

I ordered a double-double coffee and went back outside. I couldn't believe how beautiful everything was. These multidimensional beings were out enjoying the downtown area while everyone else was working. I couldn't wait to be a part of that, but I did need to get back to work. I called Hannah and asked her if she would pick me up downtown. She reminded me we were supposed to get lunch together, but she fell asleep. I assumed that higher level beings made her fall asleep so I would have time to realize everything happening around me. She apologized for falling asleep and agreed to come pick me up. She made it downtown about ten minutes later and took me back to the base. On the drive back she questioned how I was feeling. I shared no details about my discoveries because I knew she would want to send me to a mental unit at the hospital. That was the last place I needed to be.

We pulled up to the clinic where I worked and I got out of the car. I told Hannah I would see her in a little while. I didn't realize at the time that I wouldn't be home until the next morning. I went inside and made my way to the pharmacy. I took off my jacket and got right back to work. I placed my red coffee cup in my workstation so anyone coming to the window would know that I was of a higher dimension as long as they knew what to look for. Nothing extraordinary happened that afternoon. I spent most of the remainder of the day just checking prescriptions and handing out medication. I was closing the pharmacy so everyone left at 3:30 pm, but I was to stay until 4:00 pm. When 4:00 pm came around though, I couldn't get myself to leave. I felt like I had to stay behind and serve some sort of a higher purpose.

I looked in the fridge in the pharmacy to see if there was any food. Someone had left their lunch behind. I assumed that they had intentionally left it for me knowing I would be staying back with work to do. I heated it up and brought it to my office to eat. After I finished, I locked up the pharmacy and investigated the building. I knew there was something that I had to find. I just didn't know what I was looking for. The longer I stayed in the building, the stranger my thoughts became. No one else was left in the building so I believed that I was quarantined. The entire military knew I was there but didn't want to disturb me. They knew that I was a higher dimensional being and wanted me to show them how powerful I was.

I walked up and down the hallways reading the names outside of the offices. I assumed that each name represented other higher dimensional beings like myself and relished in the fact that they were here working at the base with me the whole time. They must have been watching over me. They must have been waiting for me to realize the truth. I tried to open office doors I came across, but they were all locked. Eventually I came across one that was open. It was an empty office with a computer at the main desk and a bathroom coming off of the main area. I finally found what they wanted me to find. This was supposed to be my office for the work I had to complete. The whole time I was working there, this office was ready and waiting for me and I finally realized. I wondered what work they would have for me once I got settled in.

I sat down at the computer and attempted to log in. I had to run the set up of the computer so I started the process. There was a small couch in the office to. I decided to lay down on it for a little while and soak in the fact that I finally found my purpose. I laid with my eyes closed for a couple of hours until it was dark outside. I got back up to check on the computer and the setup was complete. I could leave the computer until the next day when I had to get to work. I used the bathroom and noticed a towel hanging on the back of the door. Logically, if they set the office up for me and put a towel in it for me, they must want me to shower. I took the towel down to the second floor of the clinic and went into the male dressing room. I took off my clothes and jumped into the shower. There I was alone in the clinic of a military base showering afterhours and felt like it was normal. I felt like it was meant to be happening.

After I showered, I went down to the kitchen area and looked in the freezer. I found frozen pizzas so I heated one up in the microwave. It was delicious. I then walked around the main level for a little while looking of the medical pamphlets they had out on display. Then I thought to myself, what if they're giving me this building and the staff here to use to change the way healthcare information is delivered. They must want to combine their resources with my YouTube channel to pump out information into the masses. We could do videos on every healthcare topic and I could direct the staff here on what to do to make it a success. I felt so inspired. I would use the military to create a healthcare network. It would be perfect. I felt like this was my best idea yet.

After coming up with the idea for the military health network, I felt like my work was done and it was time to head home. I left the clinic through the bottom level doors and walked around the building. As I came up the hill to the main roadway, I analyzed the street lights. Most were orange, but some were bright white. I took this as a sign that the white lights were signals. I had to follow them as they were meant to lead me somewhere. The first building they led me to was a radar building. The radar equipment for the Navy was kept in this building. I pressed on the keypad when I got to the fence around the building and the door opened up. I notice a man walking outside near the building on the inside of the fence. I assumed he was there to lead me to where I needed to go. I followed him down the path. When we got to the end, he lit up a cigarette. I stood with him at the end of the path and we chatted briefly. When he finished his cigarette, he made his way back down the path and into the front doors of the building. I followed him in.

When I got inside, I noticed the man I followed showing his ID to security. I didn't have ID so I went up and told security that my name was Lt. Campbell and I was here to check in. They asked me if I had ID. I did not. They asked me who I was here to see. I told them I didn't know, but I was supposed to be there. I told them I was told to come there. She asked me if I could call the person who told me to come and they might clear it up. I was getting frustrated. I knew deep down this was the building where I would finally get my microchip installed, but they were making it so difficult to get in. I raised my voice and told the security guard, "I'm not leaving until someone lets me in and gets me to where I'm meant to be! I know I'm supposed to be here!" The security guard told me that if I don't have ID or know who I was there to see I would have to leave or he would be calling the police. I responded, "Whatever! Give them a call! I don't care!" I removed my smart watch and slammed it on the security desk. I then stormed out of the building. I was so frustrated. I couldn't believe they denied me access.

Just as I was venting out my frustration, I could see bright white lights overhead. I looked up and seen the penthouse of a nearby building lit up. That's where I was meant to be. I walked towards the building. I was close by so it only took me a few minutes to arrive. I walked in the doors to the hotel and approached the receptionist. I asked her if I could get a room. I gave her my ID and told her I was a veteran. I gave her my old service number for their records. She told me my room number, handed me a key card, and I was on my way. I went up to the 7th floor and found my room. When I went inside, I got in bed right away. I knew that the next day would be big since we would be starting my new health network.

I laid in bed for about ten minutes before it happened. I received telepathic communication from other worldly beings. They told me to go to the window. I got out of bed and went to open the blinds. There was a plane flying overhead on its way to the Halifax airport. I knew that someone very special was on that plane and that they were coming to see me. I looked around the room for any hints. "There was no way that this room was given to me at random. There must be something here," I thought. I opened the drawer of the bedside table and found a bible. My heart raced. I had butterflies. Could this mean that I was God? Is this why I have special abilities? Is this why I can receive messages from other dimensions? It made me wonder on the plane to come see me. I assumed one person had to be Justin Trudeau. It would make sense for the leader of the country to come and see God walking on Earth. People had written about the return of Christ, but I was confused as to why I was chosen. Was I always God or did he just choose me recently to live through? I had so many questions.

I decided in my mind at that moment that everyone I had ever met must have known that I was God. They were playing stupid or were just waiting for me to come of age and accept my place as Christ. I thought of all the hardships in my life. It made sense why I was chosen. I thought of how hard is must have been for my mother not to tell me while she was dying. It must have been torture for her to know that she would never get to see the great things I would do once I realized. I cried. The pain was excruciating. I felt as though I could feel my mother's pain and was taking it from her to deal with myself. I wished that I could see her, but I lost my ability to see the dead since I last saw her in my bedroom at the cottage during the summer of 2014. I chose at that moment, I would put on a show for the world when the sun rose.

I left my room, walked down the hall, and got into the elevator. I took it all the way to the top floor. I brought the bible with me. When I got to the top floor, I exited the elevator and opened the doors to the penthouse area. I knew the area well because we used to go there for soup at 10:00 am on Wednesdays. It was a two-story room with glass windows extended from the floor all the way to the ceiling. You could see a 180-degree view of Halifax and it overlooked the harbor. This would be perfect for when the sun rose. I would be able to see it clearly. I went upstairs to the second level of the penthouse, sat on the couch, and read the bible. I was looking for the perfect couple of versus to get my message across.

I sat there for hours until the sky lightened up. I took off my shirt and stood in the upper balcony inside the penthouse. Then it began. I screamed bible verses at the top of my lungs. I had to yell loud enough so the entire city could hear me. I knew that the room was bugged so I wanted to make it clear that I wasn't messing around. I yelled even louder. I wanted the whole world to hear me recite the verses. I was flexing my muscles and holding my arms out to the sides while I screamed. I felt so powerful. Finally, Christ has come back to Earth and his spirit was in me. I was finally recognized as a God. I stood there shouting for several minutes before I looked to my left and saw two police officers coming up the stairs towards me.

I instantly stopped what I was doing and sat back down on the couch. I put my hands in my pants pockets so they wouldn't be scared that I would try and fight. "Garrett? Garrett Campbell? How are you doing, buddy?" One cop asked. "I'm doing fine. I just really want to be left alone. I have guests coming," I responded. "Garrett, would you mind putting your shirt on and coming with us? Your girlfriend has been looking for you all night and she's really concerned for you. We all think it's best if you're checked out at the hospital." I wanted to cry. I didn't want to go back to the hospital again. It was such a painful place to be. I listened to them, though. I put my shirt back on and walked down the stairs between them. There were two paramedics waiting for us on the first level of the penthouse. They all escorted me down to ground level and put me into the back of an ambulance.

One nurse gave me some water and asked to check my blood pressure. While she put the cuff on me, I could only imagine how excited she was to be taking God's vitals. It must have been an exciting time for her. It was something she would tell all of her friends and family about. She finished checking and told me everything looked good. I nodded at her, but I refused to look into her eyes. I already knew she was multidimensional and didn't need eye contact to confirm. I also wanted no one to look into God's eyes.

The ambulance moved out of the parking lot and I got anxiety. I was concerned at what sort of tests they would want to run on me. It would be the first time they had a living God in their care. I was sure that they would be running tests for hours – maybe even days. I was ready, though. I accepted the fact that it needed to be done. I just wanted to be treated fairly. It only took us a few minutes to get to the hospital as the base was close by. When we got there, we pulled into the ambulance terminal and they took me out of the ambulance. I walked through the double doors and into a long hallway. They brought me into my own room and told me to please wait for a nurse to come see me. I waited for about 15 minutes and then a nurse entered the room. She sat down and asked me routine questions. I figured I had to play along and pretend I had bipolar disorder so I told her, "Look, I have bipolar disorder and I take Lithium for it. I've been hospitalized twice already and usually I stop taking my medication. This time I'm on it so I don't know what to tell you." She confirmed with me, "So you accept your diagnosis and know what's going on?" "Yes," I replied.

I assumed that they needed me to say the right thing so that if anyone looked into my file, it would just appear that I'm a normal crazy person and nothing extraordinary was going on. I could say nothing about being god. The nurse told me to hang out for a bit and that a doctor would come see me soon. Once she left the room, I became nervous about the whole situation. I was sure that they knew I was God, but I was stressed out about the possibility of them not acknowledging it and putting me back in the mental health unit. I didn't want to be trapped there for another 30 days. I waited for ten minutes then I had enough. I didn't want to risk going back there. I stood up and opened the door to the room I was in. I noticed the same sign as before – Staff Only. Instead of going down that road again I just looked for the nearest Exit sign and followed it. On my way down the hall. A nurse told me I had to stay here, but I just brushed her off and picked up the pace. I followed the exits signs until I was out a final set of door and outside. I was free.

As I walked towards the side walk, I felt as though I had reached an even higher dimension than before when I was downtown. I could hear the birds chirping loudly and the sun was shining bright. The air was crisp. I figured this higher dimension was a prettier version of the place I was used to living. I didn't have a jacket so I walked towards my home quickly. As I walked home, there didn't seem to be as many people around. Only a few people were on the sidewalks and there were very few cars on the road. It could have meant only one thing. Each time you ascend to a higher dimension, there are less and less people there because you leave behind everyone that hasn't made it to that dimension yet. I was fascinated by my discovery. I thought though - Maybe Hannah was gone. Maybe she didn't ascend with me. I had to get home to see if she was still there. I picked up my pace and walked as fast as I could.

When I made it to the base, I cut through as it would save a little bit of time. I entered though the East gate and made my way to the North gate. As I approached the North gate, I notice there was a Regional police car parked there. I got a pit in my stomach. I knew they were there for me. I tried to walk by without them noticing me, but when I got close to the exit, they got out of the car. "Excuse me, buddy. Are you Garrett Campbell?" One of them asked. I had to be honest. It was a rule of the higher dimensions. "Yes." I responded. "Did you just leave the hospital before seeing a doctor?" He continued. "I did, yes." He then asked, "Would you mind coming back with us so you can get checked out?" I nodded my head and walked over to the car. They put me in the back seat and we made our way back to the hospital.

When we arrived, they brought me right back to the same room. The nurse came back in and said, "You decided to go for a little walk, did you?" "Caught me," I said jokingly. She asked me if I would stay this time. I told her I would, but I was lying. There was no way I was wasting any more time sitting in the hospital. The moment she left the room, I got up and opened the door. This time I knew I had to go somewhere I wouldn't be seen by my nurse. I went the opposite way down the hallway, under the Staff Only sign and through the doors to the ambulance terminal. I left though an opened garage door. This time I knew I couldn't walk because the police would be out looking for me. I flagged down a cab and told him the address to my apartment. He took me to my building and I ran upstairs to get money and came back down to pay him. I scurried back inside was went inside my apartment. I locked the door behind me.

I ran into the kitchen and was amazed that Hannah was there. She had ascended with me. She gave me a hug and asked me where I was. I told her I got a hotel room at the base because I was scared that she would try and take me to the hospital. Then I lied and told her I was just checked out by a doctor and they let me go. She was confused as to why they let me go but was happy that I was checked out by someone. She told me she was scared when I didn't come home and made me promise never to do that again. I promised her and I meant it.

I was only home for what seemed like a moment and we heard a knock on the door. We went to open it and there was a female police officer standing there. She asked if my name was Garrett Campbell. I told her it was and she explained why she was there. "Hi, Garrett. I understand that you were at the hospital twice today to be checked out, but you left both times. Can you explain why you keep leaving?" I calmed myself and explained. "I have bipolar disorder and my doctor told me that the first thing to go before an episode is sleep. I didn't sleep at all last night so I'm scared that if I stay up any longer, something bad might happen. I left the hospital so I could come home and sleep. I was just explaining this to my girlfriend." She then asked Hannah if she was threatened. Hannah told her she wasn't. The Police officer continue to share her concerns. "We're concerned because you were found at the military base this morning acting out and you really seemed like you needed some help. If you promise that you'll stay here and get some rest then I guess I can leave you be. You seem like you're doing fine right now." I promised her I would get some rest and she left the apartment.

I felt like I had dodged a bullet. I knew I was one wrong sentence away from being taken back to the hospital again. There was no way they would have let me leave for a third time. I was so pumped up that she left me alone. Hannah asked if I would actually get some sleep now and I told her I was actually lying to the police officer; I did sleep last night at the hotel. I told her I just needed a convincing story for the police. Hannah said ok but told me to stay at the apartment and not to go anywhere. She had to go back to bed because she was working night shift later.

I kept my promise for the entire day and stayed inside the apartment. Once Hannah left for work though around 9:30 pm, I got dressed in my new outfit from the day I bought the BMW and left. I got into my car and drove it down to the military base. I showed my ID at the front gate and I was granted access. I drove to the building with the penthouse and parked. When I went inside of the building, I could hear music coming from upstairs. I followed the sounds and found a party going on. I entered the party and it was all people aged around 65 to 75. They had snacks and some were drinking. I got a beer at the bar and join them. I talked to some and realized quickly that they were all military veterans. They told me stories from their deployment's years ago. They said that they haven't seen someone my age at their gatherings before, but they liked that I was interested in hanging out with them.

As I talked to more and more of them, I developed a theory they were all war heroes and could morph back to their younger selves when the clock struck midnight. I was convinced of it. Why else would people their age be partying so hard? One of them was playing the piano and everyone else gathered around them singing as loud as they could. I was actually having a great time. I got nervous about what would happen when they all morphed. Some women were being flirty with me throughout the night. I was wondering if I was expected to have sex with them. What would be in it for me if I did? I would not be able to go through with it because I wanted to bring Hannah with me through the higher dimensions and she was my main focus. I kept singing with them until I seen someone enter back into the party from a room behind a set of tall wooden doors. I knew right away that I was meant to go in.

I made my way through the crowd and opened the doors. When I entered the room, I could see a television on a stand at the far side. I approached it and notice there was a box next to it that was full of cords. I had finally found what I was meant to find. I thought of a television show called The Black Mirror and realized that if I could just set up this television and put it on the right setting, I would finally be transported to the final dimension and be free.

I ripped the cords out of the box and untangled them. I plugged some into the back of the television and then into the wall. I turned on the television, but it was all static. I had to figure out the right channel. I flipped through a few, but each was just more static. I was becoming frustrated. Why couldn't I figure it out? I knew that I was exactly where I needed to be. After a few minutes of trying, two men came into the room and approached me. They told me I couldn't be in that room and that I would have to leave immediately. I looked at them in the eyes and told them I was supposed to be in there and that they wouldn't understand why if I told them. They repeated themselves telling me I had to go. I told them that the only way they were getting me out of the room was by dragging me out. I was much bigger than them so they became intimidated and told me that if I would not leave, they would have to call the cops. I told them to go ahead; I couldn't leave. I could tell they were frustrated, but they left the room.

I continued to mess around with the television, but I couldn't figure out how to open the portal to the final dimension. No matter what I tried, it just wouldn't work. Eventually, I heard the doors open again and this time when I turned around there were police standing behind me. I turned off the television and reached out my hands to be cuffed. They told me they weren't there to arrest me. They just wanted to help me. They knew my name was Garrett Campbell and knew that I was found in the penthouse that morning. They informed me they just wanted to make sure I received the help I needed from the hospital and asked if I would go with them to be checked out. I knew that I ultimately didn't have a choice so I nodded and acknowledged that I would come willingly. I followed the cops out and when we went through the double doors, everyone was standing in a crowd watching me being taken out. I gave them a bow and told them I hoped they were enjoying the show. We walked down the stairs, exited the building and they put me in the back of the police car.

We drove for a few minutes to the hospital and we got out of the car. When they took me inside, I went right to the same private room again and they left me alone to wait for the doctor. After a few minutes, I figured I would leave again like the last two times I was there. I exited the room, walked down the hall and left the hospital. This time though, after taking just a few steps outside, a police car turned on its lights and the cops jumped out of the car. They knew I would try and leave again. I dropped down to my knees and put my hands on the back of my head. I believed that they would shoot me. I heard them yell it was ok and I wasn't in danger. They reminded me they only wanted to get me help. They got me to my feet and brought me back to my private room. This time they cuffed me to the bed and reminded me once more that this was for my own good.

I was visited by a physician soon after and they explained that they heard about my encounter with the police at the military base and knew that I had a diagnosis of bipolar disorder. The asked me what medication I was using. I told them I was only on Lithium and that I forgot my last couple of doses. They asked if I had been using any drugs. I admitted that I had been smoking cannabis. After our conversation, they informed me they thought it was best to admit me to the mental health unit to figure out a better course of medication and try to squash the mania I was experiencing. I agreed to go to the unit and gave them Hannah's phone number. I asked them to call her and let her know where I was. They agreed that they would let her know and they went to get the police to un-cuff me from the bed. I followed a group of nurses and security up to the unit and once I got in, they had a dose of olanzapine waiting for me. I took the dose and was feeling sleepy just 30 minutes later. They brought me to bed and I passed out.

I spent the next 30 days in the unit. It was very similar to my previous hospitalizations in the sense that initially, I felt like everything was a test and that the staff were all actors. I read my horoscope from the newspaper every day for the first two weeks thinking it was a special message for me from higher beings. I also thought that my medication was a special pill to help me adjust to being in a higher dimension. These thoughts faded away halfway through my stay, though, as the medication got rid of the mania I was experiencing. The doctors added Lurasidone to my medication regimen to give me some extra coverage on top of the Lithium and they told me I would have follow up with a bipolar specialist when I got out. I also had more visitors this hospitalization. Aside from Hannah, the pharmacy staff from work also came to visit me. I was happy about that as it made me feel like I was part of the team despite no longer being a military member. I didn't attempt any escapes and I didn't kick down any doors. It was a quiet hospitalization.

EPISODE 4

AFTER THE 30 DAYS, I WAS RELEASED FROM THE UNIT. I HAD AN appointment with the specialist right away and he cleared me to go back to work. He made no adjustments to my medication but said that we may change things up down the line after we give it some time and see how I do with the new medication added. We both agreed that it was a good idea to have a mood stabilizer and antipsychotic on board.

I went back to work on a Tuesday and took things slow for my first shift. I worked at the front of the line so another pharmacist could do the prescription checks and I would just counsel patients on their medication for the first half of the day. I felt good to be back with the team and just feel normal again. It's always hard after an episode to deal with the thoughts about the way I was acting and the things I was thinking, but being back in a regular routine made a huge difference. I remember during the morning, the commanding officer of the clinic walked by the pharmacy and looked at me. She did a double take as if she was surprised to see me. She no doubt would have heard about me being found on base and was probably concerned to have me back. It made me feel awkward, but all I could do was go about my day and do my job. I was back under the direction of a bipolar specialist so I figured everything would be ok.

Later that evening, though, I got an email which made me think that things were anything but ok. My employer, sent me an email informing me that my services would not be required in the pharmacy the following day and that they would reply to me shortly with further instructions. I didn't have to wait for another email to know what was coming. I knew the state of how people with mental illnesses were treated. I had lost my position in the Canadian Forces so losing a job was nothing new. There are always commercials on television and fundraisers about breaking the stigma, but when it comes down to it, no one cares.

On Thursday, I got another email. The contracting company was informing me that my position at the base was terminated effective immediately and that I would have to meet with the regional representative on Friday to give back my key to the pharmacy and collect my things. I was no longer welcome on the base. The military informed the Nova Scotia College of Pharmacists about my illness and told them they were concerned about my capacity to practice pharmacy. I was absolutely crushed. I felt betrayed by the military. I couldn't believe that they would actually terminate someone's position based on a mental illness after the mental health campaigns I had seen them put on over the years. It was one thing to have me medical released since I couldn't be deployed but to terminate a civilian position based solely on mental health blew my mind.

I met with the regional representative the following day to return my key. She was in tears while she apologized. She seemed as shocked as I was. I knew it wasn't her company's decision so I was nothing but polite with her. I thanked her for the opportunity and was on my way back home. I thought about the position I was in. I had debt from the spending I had done while manic, I just bought a BMW, Hannah and I had rent to pay at our apartment, and I was out of a job. I knew the depression would come for me soon. I was nervous I might finally kill myself this time.

I got on the phone with veteran's affairs once I got home and filled them in on the situation. They informed me that after a medical release, Veteran's Affairs can cover up to the 90% of a veteran's salary for two years after the release date. I still had time remaining on this so they said that they would activate it soon. I was grateful that they had that program in place. This meant that I could still pay my bills and everything wouldn't fall on Hannah. I was happy to get some good news.

My positivity only lasted a few moments, though. After I got off the phone with Veteran's Affairs, I got an email from the Nova Scotia College of Pharmacists. They said that the Canadian Forces have logged a complaint against me with the college. They said that they were concerned about my capacity to practice pharmacy and that the college would have to launch an investigation. I was not to practice pharmacy until I had a meeting with representatives from the college. They gave me a number to contact and instructed me to contact them.

Before I made the call. I walked out on to our balcony. I didn't feel like I was going through a bout of depression, but the suicidal thoughts came forward in my mind. I looked over the edge at the ground. It would be so easy to step over the railing and jump. All of my problems would go away. I wouldn't have to deal with thinking about the military turning their back on me. I wouldn't have to think about losing two jobs due to mental illness. I could even stop questioning why I thought I was God and why my mind was so messed up. Like before, I couldn't get the thoughts out of my mind, though, of how much it would affect my family for something to happen. Our family can't handle another loss. I would have to go through the process and hope everything worked out better then it had been.

I went back inside and called the College of Pharmacists. During the call they explained that the complaint was regarding my mental health and that I did nothing wrong. They told me that, however, since they didn't have a specific process for people in my position who did nothing wrong, I would have to go through the same process as everyone else. This meant that I would have to go through the same process as people who steal narcotic medications from pharmacies. I would be treated the same as people who commit a crime because I have a diagnosis of bipolar disorder. They informed me also that a part of the process is having a meeting with a forensic psychologist. I was very appalled by the conversation. I felt like I was being penalized for something that was out of my control. I couldn't believe that military called the college let alone terminated my position.

I tried my hardest to stay optimistic and driven. I knew that if I sat around, I would take a deep dive into depression. I purchased a Medical Cannabis Educator Certification course and a course that allows pharmacists to order lab tests. I thought it would be good to have these on my resume for when Hannah and I eventually move home to Sydney and I'm looking for a job. I knew deep down that nothing would come out of the investigation because no errors were made and no crimes were committed. They were simply going through the process because they had to appropriately respond to all complaints that make it to the college. I spent my time working through those courses, working out in the building's gym, and adding videos to my YouTube channel.

My YouTube channel did turn into somewhat of a blessing for a little while because it gave me something to do that was pharmacy related. It was a good way to review medications while I wasn't working. After making about 20 videos however, YouTube changed their rules so you needed 1000 subscribers to be monetized. I decided to just let me channel sit and come back to it when it hit the 1000 mark.

About a month after the initial call, I had my meeting with the College of Pharmacists. Hannah came with me and we were sat in a room with the coordinator of the investigation. She went through a list of questions and all of my answers were recorded so a team of pharmacists could listen later. About halfway through, Hannah broke down and cried. She explained that I had been through so much already with my diagnosis and that it didn't seem fair to go through this process. The coordinator assured us I did nothing wrong so a decision would most likely be favorable and that we had nothing to worry about. We continued on and finished the questioning. She mentioned at the end that now that this stage was complete. I was able to work but I would have to inform whoever is hiring me about my diagnosis before working. This meant I was still unable to work. No one would hire me if they knew I had bipolar disorder. I had lost two jobs because of it and wasn't looking to lose an opportunity next. She also mentioned that I would get a call soon about my appointment with the forensic psychologist. We thanked her for her time and left the college.

The next few months were very tough for me. I felt like I didn't have much of a purpose. My time at the base was over and I wasn't able to apply for a new job because of the restriction put on me by the college. Hannah was working 10 pm to 8 am still so unless it was her week off, I didn't have much to do. I got through it without experiencing a major bout of depression. I was used to the fact that I had bipolar so I wasn't letting it get me down as much as after other episodes. I knew it was an illness and all I could do was take my medication so I did just that. I worked out here and there and finished my courses I was working on. I just wanted to get to the point to where we were ready to move home and find jobs. I knew that everything would be better once I was home around family.

We went home to visit family in December for Christmas and one day on the way from my father's place to my sister's, we drove past a home for sale. My father's place was only two blocks away from my sister's so that meant this house was close to my family. We went to take a look at it the next day. I wanted it before we even went inside just because of the location, but Hannah said she would have to renovate parts of it if she bought it. I agreed instantly. Now we just had to come up with money for a down payment. When we got back to our apartment in Halifax after the holiday, it was like a prayer was answered. When I opened the mailbox there was an envelope from Veteran's Affairs. I opening it up to find a check for $18,000. I had submitted a form a while back that was an application for a disability benefit from the military and they ruled it as favorable. It was like it was a sign we were supposed to get that house. We both agreed that we would go after it if it was still available when we were ready to move in April. A couple days later, I got an email from the College of Pharmacists that the investigation had ended and I was able to go back to practicing pharmacy. Everything seemed to work out.

Hannah kept working her job at Shoppers until April came around and we drove down to Sydney to make an offer on the house. After going back and forth a little bit we settled on a price of $194,000. The house was ours. After we had an offer accepted, I made a big mistake. To celebrate, I smoked a joint with my father. He was so happy that I was moving home so I figured it would do no harm to have a joint with him. After my first couple of puffs, I had business ideas again. I thought of an idea to use my Medical Cannabis Certification to start a cannabis educator business. I rushed out of the basement where we were smoking it and jumped onto the computer. I did up logos for what the brand could look like.

I envisioned having an office where I could educate people on medical cannabis and help them get it prescribed by a physician. I could create courses for patients and healthcare workers and sell them online. I could even go to people's houses to do a presentation. Everything was coming so fast. I stayed up late that night brainstorming.

The next day I had calmed down but I told Hannah about my idea and she actually thought it was good. People would probably be opened to learning about it from a pharmacist. I thought I was onto something. I could feel my energy level rising. I thought nothing of it, though. I just thought I was excited about a good business idea. I didn't think I was moving back towards mania. It made sense that the stress of buying a house and smoking some weed would be enough to start things though.

The house was due to close at the end of April so we closed the house and then went back to Halifax to load up a moving truck. The move went smooth and we brought everything back and unloaded it into the basement. Renovations were scheduled to start right away. Hannah had a couple of more shifts left at her store in Halifax so she went back to Halifax to finish and I stayed back in Sydney at my father's. It was probably a mistake to stay with him because we used to always smoke weed together and it was likely that we would again, but I didn't have anything set up in my new house and renovations were underway.

Just as one may have guessed. My father and I smoked weed together again. Each time, my excitement towards my business idea would grow. I was so sure of it I registered the business and posted pictures of the brand on social media. Someone from a local newspaper caught wind of it and asked me to do an interview with him. I told him I would but scheduled it for a few weeks away. I contacted my financial advisor and set up a meeting with him. I told him I would most likely be getting a massive sponsor and that I wanted him to manage the account once it gets going. He asked me about how I planned to make money with it and I had an answer for all of his questions. He was a friend besides just being my advisor so after our meeting I asked him to come out to the mall with me. When we got to the mall I spent like a maniac. We went into the jewelry store where I bought two watches. I bought some clothing and even got an item engraved with the business logo on it. The business was already making money and I was spending it.

We left the mall with bags of new items and I made my way home. When I got home, I rolled a joint and went down into the basement to smoke it by myself. I had a game on my phone I was playing and it had in-app purchases available. After I smoked, I felt like I had to beat the game right then and there. I went to the item list you could purchase and bought packages that would move you further ahead in the game. The most expensive package was $149.99. I bought it twenty times in a row and spent $3000 on my credit card. I beat the game and left the basement. When I got upstairs, I went on the computer and got the idea to share knowledge of my business on LinkedIn. When I logged in to make a profile, an offer came up for LinkedIn Premium. I instantly purchased a yearlong subscription for $650. I felt like I was making ground towards my business even though nothing tangible had happened with it. I didn't have a website, I didn't have clients, and I didn't have an office. Everything was in my head, but it felt like a reality.

About an hour after making my LinkedIn profile and setting my job description as CEO of CANN-ED Cape Breton, I got a called from someone offering me a membership to Pinnacle. They said they were associated with Forbes and that they were a network for CEOs. I felt so honored. I felt like my hard work was finally being recognized. I told her I was 100% interested and she said that all it would take was a onetime payment of $1000. I told her to hang on just a moment while I got my credit card. I gave her the number and I was all signed up. She said they would be mailing me out a package and there were forms to fill out. I thanked her enthusiastically and ended the call.

I spent the rest of the day going back and forth from the basement smoking joints to the computer thinking of more ideas for my business. I went to bed around midnight and forgot to take my medication. I slept little that night, but I did eventually fall asleep after the weed wore off and I wasn't so hyped up. When I woke up the next day, I got out of bed early. I went for a walk around Sydney and took pictures of myself and posting them to social media. There wasn't really much of a point to the pictures; I just felt the need to post them. After walking around for about two hours. My brother-in-law drove by me slowly and yelled over, "Hey, Garrett, you want a drive?" He later told me that my sister had sent him out to look for me after seeing my pictures on Facebook. When I got in the car, I was excited to see him. I instantly told him all about my business idea and how much money I would make from it. I told him that one of the large cannabis companies would become a sponsor. He played along and brought me back home. He looked at me in the eyes and asked me if I was feeling all right. I told him I was fine and that I was just excited about the business. I got out of the car and went inside.

My brother-in-law went home and filled in my sister and she called Hannah to make a plan. They both agreed that I was manic and had to get me to the hospital. They got in touch with some of my friends and told them to get me to meet them at my new house. They could just say they wanted to see it and I would go down to show it to them. Melissa and Hannah both agreed that I wasn't so far gone that the police needed to be involved. They also thought it would be embarrassing for me to get taken into a police car in the neighborhood where I just purchased a new home. My friends messaged me asking to see the house and I went down to meet them.

When I got down to the house, there was five of my close friends waiting for me. I kind of felt like something was up, but I took them inside anyway. When we got inside, they explained that they were concerned about the way I was acting. They saw the posts I was making on social media and they said that it was very uncharacteristic of me. I took offense to what they were telling me and tried to reassure them I was just excited about a new business idea. I told them I would tone it down on the posts if it would make them feel better. Then they informed me that my sister and Hannah were also very concerned. They admitted that it was actually them that wanted me to get checked out at the hospital but that they all agreed it needed to happen. Whenever I'm manic and someone wants to get me help, I always feel a sense of betrayal. I always assume that the people trying to help me don't believe in my ideas and are trying to sabotage them. I did have a strong sense of betrayal at that moment and felt like Hannah and my sister didn't care about me. I couldn't see things clearly.

I eventually agreed to go with them to the hospital so we left my house and got into one of their cars. On the way to the hospital I was telling them that this was just a big misunderstanding and that they would understand once my business gets going. They would see I had good reason to be excited. I was sure of it. When we pulled up to the hospital, I got some anxiety. I remembered my first hospitalization and how long of a stay it felt like. I didn't want to go through that again. As we got out of the car and walked inside, my anxiety only grew. With my anxiety, came irritability. My brother met us at the hospital just as we were going inside and he took me to the triage desk.

When I sat in the chair, they did the regular routine. They took my pulse, blood pressure, and temperature and then asked what we needed assistance with. My brother piped up and told the triage nurse I was experiencing a manic episode and needed to see a doctor. I chimed in and spoke aggressively, "He THINKS I'm having a manic episode, but I'm really not. I just started a new business and my friends just don't understand how huge it's going to be. Once I get it going, they'll see how big of a misunderstanding this is." My brother continued to answer her questions and I sat there disgusted listening to the conversation. She eventually told us to take a seat in the main waiting area.

It wasn't long sitting in the waiting area until I thought about how I could get out of there. I starting telling my brother that the best thing for me was to go home and take some medication. I expressed this whole process would take hours and that I wouldn't be able to sleep for a long time. I needed to take medication and sleep as soon as possible and the only way I can do that is to go home. He wasn't buying it and it frustrated me. I sat for another ten minutes thinking about what another hospital stay would be like and I just couldn't get myself to accept that I would need to do it. I eventually stood up and told everyone that I was leaving. I walked towards the doors, pushed them open and left the hospital. My brother went right to the triage nurse, told her I left and asked her to call the police to get me back in there.

When my friends came outside, I was standing at the sidewalk just outside of the hospital trying to get a taxi. They tried to express that they were just trying to help and that they needed me to go back inside, but I felt like they were doing anything but trying to help. I kept looking at each one of them in the eyes and saying, "Do you want to help me? Then leave me the fuck alone!" They didn't let up, though. They kept cutting me off when I tried to walk away and when a taxi pulled up, they would tell them we didn't need one anymore. They kept me busy long enough for the police to show up and ask me what was going on. I told them that my friends thought I was having a mental breakdown, but it was really them that needed help. I explained that I was just trying to start a business, but every time I do, my friends and family do whatever they can to ruin it. The police finally spoke up, "Listen. Your friends and your brother are concerned about you and honestly, you do seem really hyped up right now. Why don't we just go back inside of the hospital, see a doctor, and have all of this cleared up." Once the police gave me directions, I instantly complied like I always did. We went back inside as a group and the triage nurse said that they have a room ready for me. I went through a set of doors and was directed into a treatment room. They left me alone in the room and all of my friends stayed back in the waiting area with my brother. The police didn't stay with me either. I knew that if I stayed in the room, I would be looking at another 30 days in the hospital so I instantly planned my escape. I could see all of my friends through a window to the waiting room. I knew I had to get out when they weren't looking or I would probably be caught right away. I needed to find an exit, though, and I didn't know which way it was.

When a nurse came by, I asked her if I could use a washroom. She took me to the bathroom and on the way, I spotted an exit door. I went inside and pretended to use the toilet. When I came out the nurse was still waiting for me and she brought me back to my room. I then looked at the guys and waited for an opportune moment. I could see them laughing and they all looked distracted. For a moment I could see them all looking away. I slipped out of the treatment room and walked towards the exit. I slowly opened it hoping no alarm would go off. Nothing happened. I slid out the door and closed it behind me. I walked through the back parking lot and onto a dirt trail that led to a nearby reserve. About 5 minutes later and halfway down the trail, I could hear the police shouting, "There he is! Get him!" they were running after me. My instinct was to run into the woods, but I did nothing to make the police's job difficult. I always listen to them.

I stopped walking and let them catch up to me. They grabbed me by the arms and said, "Come on big guy, you know you can't be leaving like that." They brought me back into the hospital and back to my treatment room. I became very irritable. I could feel the hospital stay coming. The police cuffed me to the bed so I couldn't leave again and I yelled stuff at them like, "Oh you think you're so tough with me cuffed to the bed! Great job guys!" I also called the policeman "little man." He didn't like that. He came into the room and tightened up the cuffs. When he left the room, my uncle stepped in. He had just arrived at the hospital and wanted to see me. He asked me how I was doing and I told him I was pissed off. I didn't understand why every time I tried to start a business, people kept trying to stop me. He explained, "Starting a business is often times an early sign of going manic and your behavior usually seems erratic. It would be totally fine to start a business, but we get concerned when you start acting this way."

I felt trapped and my irritability increased. I had delusional thoughts. I told my uncle that the real reason I'm at the hospital is because people were trying to stop Hannah and I from getting into our house and eventually get married. My uncle tried to clarify with me, "You think you're in the hospital because you and Hannah got a house?" I responded, "You know it's the truth, Lucas." He tried to re assure me that no one was trying to stop Hannah and me from living together, but I wasn't listening to him. I knew it to be true in my mind.

Eventually a doctor came to see me and it didn't take him long to decide to admit me to the mental health unit. I felt overwhelmingly betrayed as I followed the nursing staff down the hall to the unit. It was the last place I wanted to be. It turned out not to be completely the right place for me either. Since my last time being in the unit, they got a computer set up with internet. I got on Facebook and posted more about my business from inside the hospital only to make my embarrassment even worse post hospitalization.

This episode was good in other ways, though. My family got me to the hospital while I was still in the early stages of mania and I didn't start having delusions about being God or everyone being actors. I didn't think about multi-dimensional beings or having special abilities. Once they saw the signs of starting a business and being erratic about it, they jumped on it and got me help. They did a great job. Unfortunately, I would become better at keeping to myself during my final episode and would experience severe delusions and hallucinations.

THE FIFTH EPISODE

I GOT OUT OF THE HOSPITAL WITH A NEW MEDICATION REGIMEN.
I still had the lithium on board, but the psychiatrist added Zeldox
(ziprasidone) to it. He thought it would give me better coverage than what
I was taking before. It was a newer agent. I committed to taking it regularly
and prayed that it would work for me. I felt a lot of embarrassment
following my fourth episode because I could remember acting like a
lunatic in front of my friends. They understood that it was part of the
illness, but it's just hard when I can remember the details about how I
was acting. I couldn't understand what made me think those thoughts
and act that way. The renovation was about two months away from being
complete when I got out of the hospital so we stayed at my father's place
until it was ready.

We moved in on August 23rd and my best friend rented a room
from us. The first few months were great. We had people over all the
time, family would come to visit us, and the three of us would have the
odd kitchen dance party. After a couple of months, I grew concerned

about getting a job. I had been watching for postings the entire time, but there just wasn't any pharmacist positions being posted. It took until late October until I had something to apply for. Hannah's mother found a posting for a pharmacy IM/IT Business/Systems analyst with Nova Scotia Health Authority just minutes away from my house. I jumped at the opportunity to apply and was granted an interview. It turned out to be a long process but, in the end, I was hired on and I started in January.

During the same month, my YouTube channel had finally made it to 1000 subscribers and was monetized. The income was only set at $20 a month but with only 20 videos posted I seen the potential in it. Over the next few months, I posted 10 videos a week after work and quickly built it up to over $400 a month. I was proud of having a side hustle that actually worked and I liked that I was still educating people on medication after taking a non-practicing pharmacy position.

Though, my father struggled with depression and felt like he had to get out of his house. He was living in the house we grew up in alone and it was full of memories of my mother. He found the winters long and he couldn't stop thinking about her. He went to the hospital in the mental health unit because he became suicidal. This hit me hard and caused me a lot of stress. I had lost my mother and I couldn't imagine if anything happened to my father. I considered him to be one of my best friends; I couldn't lose him. I became very passionate about the situation and told my father that when he got out of the hospital, he could come live with us for a little while until he figured something out.

He was in the hospital for about 30 days until he was finally released. He was given an antidepressant and he actually agreed to take it. This was uncharacteristic for him. The next couple of months were tough having him live with us, but I knew we were doing the right thing. He would rearrange our furniture, put decorations around the house, and be waiting for me after work to drive him around Sydney when all I wanted to do was make my YouTube videos.

Eventually the stress got to me and I turned to cannabis to help calm it down. I had no symptoms of mania right away – the new medication must have delayed it – but over the coming months as my cannabis use increased, I acted a little different.

My YouTube channel was sitting at about 120 videos and I was feeling very driven. One day I decided to make three videos a day for 30 days straight. I thought it would be just the challenge my channel needed to push it over the edge. I ordered a new 4K camera for my channel. It was something I knew I needed, but I felt a little more open to spending money. I thought that I had the right drive to eventually push my channel to 100,000 subscribers. I didn't care if it took years to accomplish. I knew I would get there someday. I was working out a lot to. I had a calendar set up in my home gym and I had worked out for 60 days straight. In my mind, all I had to do was go to work, workout, and make YouTube videos and I would finally become successful.

After finishing five days of creating videos I became stressed and my anxiety spiked. I felt like my family would somehow come and try to stop me from achieving my goals. I had it engrained in my mind from previous manic episodes that whenever I try to achieve success, they come to stop me. I called my aunt and voiced my concerns to her and she tried her best to calm me down. She thought the YouTube channel was a great idea and loved that I was putting so much time into it. I still couldn't get myself to continue creating videos, though, and my anxiety slowly turned in a sense of superiority. I felt like I was above other people. This was the first sign that something was going on.

The last video I had done was actually on Zeldox, the medication I was using. In my research for the video, I discovered that when someone is using it to treat bipolar, they are supposed to be taking 40mg twice daily. I was only on 20mg once daily. I immediately called my physician's office and made an appointment. I told them it was urgent so they got me in the next day. When I got to my appointment, I was honest with my doctor. I told him I was having thoughts of superiority and that I was scared I was slowly drifting towards mania. He agreed that my dose was too low and we increased it to the recommended 40mg twice daily. By that time though, it was too late because I had developed a craving for cannabis. It was legal in Canada then so all I had to do to get it was drive to the nearest shop to pick some up. This was a recipe for disaster. I smoked it with my father while he was living with us.

The first real signs came just days later. I thought again about people around me being actors. I thought that life was just a game again. This time though, I was not in the matrix. I thought that the world was my playground. The more I thought about it, the more I realized that everyone was an actor, even my family. I thought that my mother was still alive somewhere and that she faked her own death to test me. I was experiencing the Truman Syndrome. The Truman syndrome is a type of delusion in which the person believes that their lives are staged reality shows, or that they are being watched on cameras. I felt trapped. I knew I couldn't turn to anyone for help because everyone was part of the game. I wondered if my medication was even real. Was I ever crazy in the first place? I knew that once I tried to get help, the world would come down on me and I would be sent back to the hospital only to reset the show. It would be a never-ending cycle. I knew suicide wasn't an option because once I tried to attempt it someone would interfere and this would also land me back in the hospital. I didn't know what to do.

I tried my hardest to go to bed each night and to go to work like I was supposed to do. I would try to keep my interactions at work to a minimum. I wanted no one to catch on that I knew what was going on. Luckily my new role wasn't in a social setting, the work was done on the computer. I got through each day and made it back home to where it was safe. The most difficult part was conversing with Hannah. We had recently got engaged in November, but I didn't know if she loved me. There was a possibility she could have fallen in love with me after being given the role of my girlfriend, but I knew she was planted in the right place at the right time for us to meet. How could I live my whole life with someone knowing she was just playing a role?

After a few days of going to work and coming home to work out, I got used to living my life in the reality show. I would try my hardest not to give the show any more outbursts and what they called manic episodes. I would try to live a boring life and make them wish they had never done this. I often wondered just how far their reach was. After thinking about the places I had travelled to in the past, I realized that it wasn't just my community but the entire world. Every single person on Earth was an actor there only to interact with me. It was an amazing revelation. If the entire world was my playground. That meant that I could do anything. I just had to stick to the rules and put on a good show. I started enjoying myself a little more.

I took Hannah out to eat more often and smoking more cannabis. Smoking cannabis helped me figure everything out to a higher degree. One night I was outside in the backyard smoking a joint and I was looking up at the stars. I thought to myself that if everyone on Earth was an actor, then someone had to be running the show. As I continued to smoke, I realized that the controllers of this show or this game must be off world. Then it hit me – It wasn't just everyone on Earth watching me - It was the entire galaxy; it was the entire universe. All of the species of aliens out in the universe were watching my every move. I stood up and waved at the stars. I knew that they weren't actually stars. They were alien spaceships circling around our planet watching me. I took out my phone and starting playing music and dancing for them. I even turned around and shook my booty at them. I wanted them to know that I could see them and that I was ok with it. I didn't mind they were watching me. I actually felt honored.

It was a Friday night so I knew I had time to figure out more about my situation. When I finished smoking my joint I went right inside and rolled another one. I put on my headphones and played music at maximum volume. I wanted whoever was watching me to think I was just having a normal night. I knew that the actors on Earth didn't know that everything was being run by aliens so I didn't want them to think I had stumbled across anything special. The music made me feel more empowered. When I walked back outside, I pointed at the stars to tell the aliens I was back and ready to chat with them more. Through smoking cannabis, I spoke with them telepathically. I grabbed a lawn chair, set it up under the stars, and gazed at the aliens while I smoked my joint.

While I was communicating with them, I started to undercover some troubling information. Everything wasn't exactly how I had imagined. Our planet was being watched by aliens, but it wasn't just me being watched. It was everyone. Earth was set up in a way that when someone uncovers the truth and unlocks their true potential, everyone else brings them back down and keeps them in line. It was a self-governing society and made sure no one got too empowered. This is why every time I came up with a new idea, my family would say it was because I was crazy and locked me up in the hospital. If everyone discovered the truth, we could live as a free planet and everyone could live to their true potential. The aliens told me it was up to me and other people like me to save the planet. I didn't know what to think. This was a massive discovery and I felt intimidated. Every time I try to do something for myself, I would get locked away and now I had to unlock everyone's potential somehow. The aliens told me I had everything I needed and that I would find a way.

I needed a break from communicating telepathically. I went inside to get some food. I would need all the energy I could get to keep up my new mission. While I was eating, I wondered why I was chosen. Maybe it was because of my military training. Maybe it was because I understood the pain of loss from when my mother passed away. I wasn't sure what the answer was, but I accepted their request and vowed to do whatever I could. I knew I had to do it from the confines of my own home, though. I could sense that everyone was just waiting to take me to the hospital. One wrong move and I would be locked away again for 30 days and I didn't know when my telepathic abilities would come back.

I finished eating and rolled another joint. I needed my abilities to be running at maximum capacity for the aliens to guide me to the right answers. They said I have everything I needed, but I still needed their assistance. Cannabis was the only thing that would ensure an open line of communication. When the joint was rolled, I went back outside to sit under the stars. I took out my phone and opened the Twitter app. I made a fake profile and looked up terms like aliens, enlightenment, and telepathic. I followed a bunch of accounts but still didn't know if I was on the right track. Then I thought about my last time in the hospital and remembered how much the horoscopes lined up with me. I looked up an account for Taurus horoscopes and followed it. I read some to make sure they still lined up. They did.

Then I remembered that the aliens told me it was up to me and people like me – not just me. I followed the other horoscopes. I needed to have the horoscopes working together. I lit up the joint for more focus. After a few puffs I quickly realized that I needed to find people on Earth who are awake that matched the 12 horoscopes. We needed the power of the stars to save Earth. I looked up Mark Zuckerberg's zodiac sign and realized that it was Taurus. I couldn't use him because I already filled that position. I checked Justin Bieber's sign. He was a Pisces. I followed him on Twitter and continued on. Next, I checked LeBron James. He was a Capricorn. I followed him on Twitter and went to the next name that came to mind. I continued to check the zodiac signs of people with a lot of influence until I had all twelve signs filled. Some other names I checked were Jeff Bezos, Elon Musk, and Warren Buffet. I checked Dwayne Johnson as well, but he was also a Taurus so he didn't make the cut.

I now had a fake Twitter account following twelve influential people of different zodiac signs. I became nervous that the militaries of the world would be alarmed at how fast I was figuring everything out. As I took my last puff of the joint, my nerves settled and I realized that the militaries were probably on my side. They would want the world to be saved. Just as I thought this, I thought I saw something moving in a window in one house surrounding my yard. I assumed it was a sniper. I got out of my chair and ran inside. Why was there a sniper watching me? It could only mean I had figured it out. They don't want me telling anyone. If I do, they'll kill me. I shut off the lights in my house so that no one could see where I was. I looked out other windows in my house and could tell that every window in sight of my house had a sniper in it. I was surrounded.

I had to think of a way to communicate with them. I knew that they were monitoring everything I owned and that the aliens told me I had everything I needed. I ran downstairs and grabbed my apple watch. I put it on my right wrist. I then went to my bedroom and grabbed my Samsung smart watch. I put that on my left wrist. I then grabbed my Samsung galaxy phone and my Apple work phone and sat on my couch. The Apple phone and watch were being monitored by America and the

Samsung phone and watch were being monitored by China. If I send messaged back and forth, it would force the two most powerful countries in the world to work together to monitor me. This would also show them that I'm being transparent. By wearing my smart watches, it would ensure that both militaries had access to my vitals. They could use that information to track how I was holding up and the tracking abilities of the phone and watches would be useful.

I felt like I got my message across so I walked over to the kitchen light switch. I closed my eyes and turned it on. I didn't get shot. That must have meant that they bought what I was selling with the devices idea. I felt like I could now walk around freely, but the snipers were still in place if I acted out of line. I had to be on my best behavior. I put my music back on and went downstairs to roll another joint. This time when I went outside, I embraced the fact that I was Taurus walking around on Earth. I was the most powerful of all the zodiac signs. This is why the military was watching me so closely. I could destroy the entire planet in the blink of an eye if I chose to. I stood in my back yard in a power pose and smoked my joint. I didn't care that the snipers were watching me. I felt confident that they were now on my side but just wanted to make sure I didn't overstep.

I thought that I should test the world I was now living in. I wanted to see if the people watching over me would help me. I decided I would find a VLT and see if they were now programmed to give me cash when I needed it. I suspected they would be a type of ATM for me. I used to work security on the nearby reserve so I figured that I could go up there to run my test. I finished with my joint, went inside, and called a taxi. I couldn't risk getting pulled over after smoking and messing everything up. The cab came quickly and I went outside and got in. I told him where I was going but asked him to stop at a store along the way. The building I was going to was for smokers so I wanted to fit in. We stopped at a store and I bought a pack of cigarettes. I was then dropped off outside of the VLT building. When I went inside, I went to the ATM and took out a single $20 bill. It was all I needed to run my test. I walked about the room looking at all of the VLTs seeing which one would catch my eye. On one of them there was a cartoon picture of a person with massive blue eyes. It was perfect. I remembered the connection of eye contact and higher dimensional beings from my previous episode. I sat down, put in my twenty and hit the Max Bet button. I broke even on the first spin so I pressed it again. I lost. I thought there must be some sort of a switch on the machine I could use for it to acknowledge it was me playing. There was a loose compartment on the bottom of the machine. I pressed my knee against it and held it in its proper position. I hit the Max Bet button three more times and bit the bonus. I was awarded 10 free spins. As they began, I pressed my knees even harder against the machine. I had to make sure that I was holding the compartment in its proper position. I watched as the money kept rolling in. I would collect more money with each free spin. By the end of the bonus round, my balance was at $132. I cashed out and went to the front cage to get my money. I went outside and lit up a cigarette. It felt so nice to know that the VLTs were programmed to give me money. Now anytime I needed funds, I could just quickly play on one and get everything I needed.

I enjoyed every puff of the cigarette I took which was uncharacteristic of me because usually I can't even handle one puff. In that moment, the cigarette was amazing. After I finished the first one, I took out a second and puffed it. When I finished, I walked to the nearest store and bought a bunch of snacks. I bought pizza burgers, energy drinks, chocolate bars, and chips. It wanted to consume everything. I felt like it was all free. I didn't need much to be happy. I knew I could have stayed at that VLT all night and won thousands of dollars, but I just needed to confirm that money was available when I needed it.

When I finished in the store, I called a taxi and went back home. When I arrived, Hannah was back from work. She asked me where I was and I told her the truth. I told her I just felt like gambling since I didn't do it in such a long time and because I was bored at home. Right away, she asked me if I was feeling ok. She said that it was unlike me to have an urge to gamble and that I smelled like cigarettes. I admitted that I had one and she turned around and stormed into our bedroom. She came back with my medication. "I need you to take this right now," she ordered. I grabbed a glass of water and took my medication like she asked. She said she had to go to bed soon because she was working at 8:00 am the next day. She told me I had to come to bed with her. I listened to her and got in bed, but the second she fell asleep, I snuck out and went down to the basement to roll a joint. I wanted to celebrate that I had infinite money at my fingertips from the programmed VLTs. I finished rolling my joint and went outside. This time while I was smoking the joint the stars moved. They were all moving slightly in little circular patterns. This was their way of telling me they were happy with my accomplishments. They were rewarding me with a little show.

I ran inside, grabbed my headphones, and blasted music. I felt like as a zodiac, I could control the stars. I reached out to them pulling them towards me. I wanted to bring them closer to Earth. I wanted everyone to see them. By pulling them closer, I was requesting their assistance in the saving of the planet. I knew that they would leave it up to me, but I wanted them to feel included in my mission. While I was doing my star work, I could feel how intimidated the snipers were becoming. This was the first time they saw someone manipulating the galaxy. Song after song, I reached to the stars and performed my manipulations. After a while I saw new stars appears. This meant that other races of aliens were becoming comfortable enough to show themselves. Different races from all over the universe were coming to the Milky Way to witness my greatness.

After I felt like I had done enough, I sat down and took out my phone. I opened up Twitter and saw that someone I was following had shared a post about Jimmy Fallon. I took it as a sign that I should follow him, so I did. Many of his tweets were about his show. I looked up the time it was starting and realized it was coming on soon. I rushed inside, turned on the television, and found the right channel. I stood directly in front of the TV while it started. Each time it showed Jimmy, I stared into his eyes trying to confirm if he was a higher being. He was. This meant that he could sense I was looking at him. I tried to see if he felt uncomfortable. He seemed alright. Could he be a zodiac like me? I quickly checked on my phone when his birthday was. He was Virgo. I had finally confirmed the first sighting of another zodiac sign on Earth. Everyone else I was following on Twitter were just my best guesses, but now I was sure I found one. I spent the duration of the entire show standing in front of the television watching his every move. He must have been given the task of entertainment. I knew each zodiac sign would have a different task, but I didn't realize even entertainment would be involved. I suspected that mine was power and using the military. That was why all the militaries of the world were monitoring my every move.

After Jimmy Fallon's show ended, another late-night show came on. I was amazed that the host of it also seemed to be a zodiac sign. I couldn't get my head around it. Why were these zodiacs performing comedy? The world needed strength, not laughter. Then I had another thought. Maybe we weren't zodiac signs at all. Maybe we were Gods. Perhaps they were trapped in their roles because it was their way of blending in and keeping themselves safe. All this time they were waiting for a God more powerful then themselves to arrive and set the world straight. I was that God. I was the God of all Gods. I was Jesus Christ. I was on Earth to fulfill the prophecy of reincarnation. I didn't know exactly why I was chosen, but I accepted it. I had to roll a joint to help figure everything out and increase my abilities.

I rolled a joint in the basement and brought it outside again. I stared up at the stars while I smoked it. I waited for the information to come. I appreciated the night's sky. I wished that I could remember creating it, but my past memories were blocked. I felt like if I consumed enough cannabis, I eventually got my memories back. As I thought about being Jesus Christ, I felt lonely. I thought I created humans so perfectly, but they seemed to have lost their way. I pondered if I had to cause a cataclysmic event to reset the planet or if I could set things right. I also felt scared. Last time I came to Earth, I was crucified. Would they accept me this time or would they torture me all over again? I had so many questions that needed answers, but I was the creator of the universe. Who could I turn to? I went back inside and sat in the dark thinking. I realized that I could only tell one person the truth about who I was. Only Hannah could know.

I stayed up all night waiting for her to get up for work and I sat her down. I explained to her I had discovered something incredible and that I didn't want her to be scared. I told her, "Hannah, there's no easy way to tell you this so I'm just going to come out and say it. I'm God. I know it sounds crazy, but it's the truth. You have to trust me on this and promise not to tell anyone." She got up, went to the bedroom and grabbed our emergency supply of olanzapine, a strong antipsychotic. She took out two pills and handed them to me. "Take these," she ordered. I felt so rejected. I couldn't understand why she wouldn't believe me. I knew I had to do what she said or she would call the police. I was scared that they would try to execute me when they arrived so I took the medication. Hannah then got on the phone and let her boss know that she would be running late to work due to a health emergency. When she hung up, she told me to put my jacket on and get in the car. We were going to the hospital. I continued to feel rejected but continued to follow her commands.

We went outside, got in the car, and drove to the hospital. We parked far away from the doors and during the walk, all I could think of was that they would never believe me. They wouldn't accept that God has returned to Earth. We slowly made our way inside and approached the triage nurse. She told me to sit down and we went through the regular process – blood pressure, heart rate, and temperature. Hannah told the nurse I have bipolar disorder and I'm experience a manic episode. After she finished giving her the details, we took a seat in the waiting room.

As I looked around the room at the people waiting with us, everything became obvious. These weren't people. They were angels that watched over me and ensure that nothing bad happened. They were just disguised as regular people. I tried to look at one of them in the eyes and they locked eyes with me just for a moment. It was all I needed to confirm my suspicion. I felt safe. After a little while, a woman sat down near us with a small child. He must have been two or three years old. The child kept looking into my eyes and didn't look away. This shocked me. It meant that he was a God like me. His mother must have brought him to show me that God's exist at all ages. I was amazed. Did the child know he was a God? Then unexpectedly, the child communicated with me telepathically and told me he read my mind and wanted to answer my question; he did know that he was a God. I felt an overwhelming feeling of contentment. I finally knew that I wasn't alone. I wondered how many God's there were on Earth. Would I be able to meet them all someday? I became concerned that if I was put in the hospital again, I would again lose my abilities and possible forget what I really am.

I then wondered why Hannah wouldn't believe me. I was also concerned about why she always became so happy when she gets me to the hospital. It was torture for me, but she seemed to smile more as I became more uncomfortable. The only thing that made sense was that our spirits were connected in a reverse duality. She could be happy only if I was in pain and vice versa. One of us had to sacrifice ourselves for the other. If I was being tortured, she would be happy. If I felt content, she might die. This must be how love works. It's impossible for both people to be completely happy. One must give up happiness. I would do that. I decided at that moment I was ready to die for Hannah. If it was the only way for her to experience true bliss. I would gladly let the world kill me because I loved her. Just as I concluded that, the child telepathically said "Now you finally understand."

I had to focus on negative thoughts. The more depressed I could become, the better Hannah's life would be. I thought of the day I watched my mother take her last breath and how I saw my father cry for the first time. I thought of the relationships I screwed up due to my immaturity. I thought of the military and how they turned their back on me when I was diagnosed with a mental illness. The negative thoughts kept flooding into my mind, but I loved it. I wanted to go to hell. Then I heard a nurse call my name. Hannah got me up and brought me out back; the nurse led us to a treatment room. When we got inside, I explained to Hannah why I wasn't allowed to be happy anymore. I told her we were connected in such a way she could be happy only if I was experiencing intense pain. I told her I could handle it and if need be, I would die for her. She smiled laughing a little bit and told me that everything would be ok. When I saw her laugh, I winced in pain. It was excruciating. I told her to look at what she was doing. She tried to hold back her laughter, but she found it funny. The more she laughed, the more pain I felt. Our spirits were now 100% connected.

A psychiatrist came into the room moments later and sat down in front of us. Hannah explained the situation to him. I knew that the psychiatrist recognized me because I saw him in the mental health unit often. During their conversation, Hannah smiled. Just as her smile took shape, I winced in pain again. The psychiatrist asked me what was wrong and I told him, "She's torturing me with her happiness. Our spirits are connected and our happiness is reversed. Only one of us can be happy. I already died for her many times." He then asked me how often I died. I said, "Infinite times. I've died every possible death known to man." He gave Hannah a look and said that he would be back in a few moments.

As he left the room, I could feel the building vibrate. The hospital gained the ability to travel through different dimensions and I was on my way to hell. I was happy that I was going there. If I was in hell, Hannah could finally live her life in heaven. The building stopped vibrating just as the psychiatrist entered the room again. He told us I would be admitted to 1B, a mental health unit. We got up and followed a nurse to the unit. When we entered, Hannah informed me she had to make her way to work. I gave her a hug and she left. The nurses brought me into a room to do an admission interview. I sat down and only one nurse stayed in the room with me. In that moment, I knew that I was only in the unit for my protection and the nurses were angels. During the interview one question was if I needed anything right away. I told her I could use a Keith's and thought she would get it for me. I imagined them there only to serve me. I kept giving bogus answers to her questions so she eventually said that we would continue the interview later. She gave me a quick tour of the unit and then left me alone.

The first thing I did was to walk into the common area where a few patients were hanging out playing cards. I scanned the room trying to look at each person in the eyes. I realized right away these were not angels.

These individuals were the people throughout my life that ever wronged me. There were members of the military, family members, and old friends. They had taken a different form to blend in. They didn't think I could see through their disguises. They wanted me to forgive them for them to be released from hell. I wanted them to stay with me so I left the room with no forgiveness. Next, I scanned the hallways, I saw a man with tattoos all over his arms. He to thought his disguise was fooling me. I knew right away that it was actually Eminem. He must have sinned and expected me to resolve them. I was a big fan so I helped him. I grabbed him by the shoulders and put my forehead against his until I could only see one large eye. It was the all-seeing eye of the illuminati. He must have gotten tangled up with them. Once it came into focus, he quietly told me to slow down. I pulled my head away and made a cross on his forehead with my thumb. Then I placed my palm on his head and shoved him away from me. He let out a loud scream. My job was done.

I could see a man down the hall walking around in circles. I ran down to him and got down on one knee. I recited the prayer Our Father. I closed my eyes and could hear his footsteps. The steps became more plentiful. I could feel an army of angels forming around me. They came to hell to give me assistance. I opened my eyes to see nurses standing around me. One of them said, "Garrett, you can't be touching patients. You're going to have to come with us." I stood up and followed them. They brought me out of the unit and down the hall to unit 1C; it was a unit for more at-risk patients. Once I walked in, I instantly calmed down. There were only three other patients in the unit I could see. It felt peaceful. I knew that if I wanted to get out in less than 30 days, I would have to play by the rules. A nurse that treated me during my first episode approached me to give me a tour of the unit.

Over the next ten days, I did everything by the book. To blend in, I even went outside with the patients in my unit to smoke cigarettes. Through going outside with them, I became friends with one patient. He told me he was diagnosed with bipolar as well, but he was actually the Devil. This confirmed my thoughts I was in hell. I told him I was God and asked him to keep it to himself. We were a match made in heaven – pardon the pun. We talked constantly about what our roles were as God and the Devil. I told him I have to take on other people's pain so they could be happy and that I loved doing it. He told me that his job was to fuck people over for his own benefit. We had many fascinating conversations. I did such a good job at playing by the rules I was released in just thirteen days.

This time being released from the hospital, I still had all of my abilities and still knew that I was God. I was released on a Sunday and went back to work the following day. I stuck to myself for most of the day trying not to let on what I actually was. I learned my lesson that any time I talk to someone about it, I would be sent to the hospital and back to hell. On my lunch break, I went home to have a few cigarettes I got from the Devil. I sat in the back yard enjoying all of my creations. I was looking at the grass in awe, taking in the blue skies, and admiring the Sun. I felt like the sun was my most beautiful creation. It was the only thing I knew of that was as powerful as I was. In that moment I felt like I should test my abilities. I should prove to myself that I am more powerful than the sun. I widened my eyes and stared directly into it. After a few seconds, I had to pull away. My eyes were burning. I shook my head and turned towards it again, staring intensely. My eyes burned again, but this time I refused to look away. I widened my eyes even more and screamed. This time when I widened my eyes, the sun rays disappeared and I could focus easily on the sun. I continued to stare. To my surprise, the sun turned black. I was causing an eclipse. What would the people of Earth think? I closed my eyes and thought to myself that I'm the most powerful being in the universe.

Just as I opened my eyes again, a plane was flying by low. I assumed that they were watching me. I stared at it and could sense that Warren Buffet and Dwayne "The Rock" Johnson were on board. They wanted to come meet me. Who wouldn't want to meet the man that could stare into the sun? I pointed at the plane and then gave a casual salute. I checked the time on my phone and realized I had to get back to work soon. I was excited to finish out the day so I could get back to testing my abilities and admiring my creations. As I walked inside, I could see that my father was standing by the window. This meant that he was also watching me. I assumed he was proud.

I made my way back to work and finished out the three-hour afternoon. Nothing eventful took place as I stayed low key. When I arrived back at home, I went right down into the basement to roll a joint. I needed to see if there was anywhere higher for my abilities to go. I brought the joint out into my sanctuary in the back yard and lit it up. As I smoked it, I realized that I wasn't thinking big enough. I thought I was on Earth to resolve the sins of humans, but I was neglecting the animals. As I thought of this, I focused on the birds as they flew by. I tried to stare into their eyes, but it was tough as they were flying by so fast. I tried again and again. I kept looking around and saw a bird sitting on a tree in my neighbor's yard. It was staying still and appeared to stare at me. I stared back. Before I knew it, it communicated with me telepathically. It told me it was also a God and that God's can take many forms. Many are cats and dogs. I was amazed. This taught me I still had a lot to learn about the higher dimensions.

I walked over to the side of my house and sat on a chair. I reached out my arms to the side hoping that a bird would come and land on me and speak for a little while. Much to my surprise, a fly landed on my hand. I slowly brought it in closer to my face. I stared into its eyes. It, like the bird, talked . He was the God of the flies and he wanted to introduce himself. I was happy to meet him. He stayed on my hand for quite a while before finally taking off and flying away.

My father came outside shortly after to hang out with me. We set up two chairs and sat side by side. He kept starting casual conversations with me, but I found it hard to relate. My head was out in the universe exploring different planets or telepathically speaking with animals as they approached the house. I couldn't enjoy talking about normal things like work or the weather. I wanted to tell him I was God so badly. I wanted him to know what I was capable of. Then I thought there was a possibility he already knew. He did raise me after all. Maybe he was waiting all this time for me to realize for myself and admit it. This seemed to make sense. I couldn't risk coming out and saying it, but in that moment, I truly believed that my father knew I was God. I had to find a different way to demonstrate it to him. This would take some thought. Meanwhile, I would just act like a human as best as I could.

I started by getting up and doing some cleaning. My garage was a mess and a lot of things had to come out now that winter was ending. I took out the gardening tools and placed them by the garden, I organized the bags of cans and bottle, and then I saw the hose. I had an idea. I hooked up the hose and brought it outside. I sprayed my lawn. I could make summer come faster if I watered the Earth. I wasn't just watering my grass; I was watering the entire Earth. I knew that Mother Nature liked when people cared for her and I could sense that the animals around me were proud. After I finished watering, I moved towards and old mattress laying on the ground outside the garage. When I picked it up, I could see that ground was covered in worms. They were everywhere. I was shocked. I looked at my father and back down at the worms. I knew that the seven great plagues were starting.

I dropped the mattress and ran inside. I went directly down to the basement and grabbed a bible off of my bookshelf. I started frantically flipping through it looking for anything I could find about the plagues. I needed to stop them. I couldn't find what I was looking for. I ran back upstairs and grabbed my phone. I had to make sure Hannah was ok. I wanted her to get home, but she was at work. I thought to myself, "Fuck it." I called her anyway. When she answered I told her I was just calling to make sure she was all right. She laughed and said she was. I then told her I was scared something bad would happen to her and was wondering if she could leave work. She instantly knew what was happening. She told me to go into the bedroom and get the olanzapine. She wanted me to take 20mg. She then told me she would call my sister, Melissa and my brother, Logan.

Logan arrived shortly after and told me that everyone was concerned with how I was acting, and that Melissa and Hannah think I was released from the Hospital too early. He said we had to go back. I asked my brother if I could have a cigarette and take a shower before we go. I think he was amazed that I agreed to go so he said that it was fine. I went outside and lit my last cigarette. I puffed it slowly and softly. It tasted perfect. I thought to myself that I was hoping the Devil would still be at the hospital so we could continue our discussion. He would probably be happy to know that the plagues were about to start and wreak havoc on Earth. He may have even initiated them. I also thought about how I wouldn't be able to see the stars while I was in the hospital. That made it more difficult for me to travel the galaxy and the universe. I took out my phone and typed in galaxy in the app store. I found an app called Galaxy Map. I opened the app and could see that our Galaxy, the Milky Way, was depicted as a plane of perfect spirals. Everything was level on the same plane except the Canis Major Overdensity. I finally knew my purpose. I had to realign it within the galaxy to save the Earth. I put my phone in my pocket and went inside to shower.

After taking as long of a shower as I could, I got dressed and was ready to. We got in the car and went to the hospital. When we went inside, we did the regular triage routine, sat in the waiting room, eventually went into a treatment room, talked to a psychiatrist, and I was admitted. They put me back in unit 1C for high risk patients. When I got inside, I became upset with the Devil. I thought initially that I would be happy to see him, but once I pictured the world crumbling under the pressure of the plagues, I lost it. I screamed at him that what he was doing was wrong and ordered him to stop. He just stood there and laughed at me. I could tell he was feeding off my frustration. A couple nurses rushed into the common room and told me to calm down. I turned to them and continued to scream, "Don't you dare tell me to calm down! Do you have any idea what I'm capable of?" I turned to the wall and punched it as hard as I could. They continued to try to calm me down, but I wasn't having it. Eventually a nurse came in with an injection. A team of nurses held on to me while one injected me in the shoulder. The medication kicked in fast and I was barely able to stand up. They walked me to my room and put me to bed.

I woke up many hours later with a headache and a dry mouth. I struggled to get out of bed but managed to after a couple of tries. I went to find the Devil. When I finally found him, I told him we had to resolve our differences. He asked me if I wanted to go outside for a cigarette. I agreed to. While we were outside, we talked about all problems with the world, but when we tried to discuss solutions we were always on opposite sides with our proposals. He wanted to kill everyone on Earth, and I wanted to awaken them. He continuously told me they weren't worth saving. I refused to agree. I knew I had the power to do it.

We talked often over the next two weeks and then eventually our conversations switched from how to deal with the world to what type of coffee we should get from Tim Hortons. We had both made our way back to baseline after many doses of antipsychotics. They kept me at the hospital for an extra two weeks to be safe and then once again, I was released. Over the next few months, I would have a few bouts of depression. My fifth episode was hard to deal with because I couldn't comprehend how my brain would produce such wild thoughts. That episode also scared me. That I was confident enough to stare into the sun messed me up. When the sun turned black, it wasn't an eclipse. It was my retina burning. I caused permanent eye damage to my left eye. If it was possible for me to stare into the sun, what would stop me from doing something like thinking I could fly and walking off a building? I was scared I would die if I continued to become manic each year. I promised myself to never miss a dose of my medication ever again and to take extra medication any time I didn't have a full 8-hour sleep. I promised myself that I would never smoke cannabis again as it clearly pushed me into mania several times. I became willing to do whatever it took to stay healthy.

It's been about two years since my last episode and I mostly just struggle with depression. I'm in a good position in life and have everything I've always wanted, but I'm scared to let myself be happy. For the last five years, I've been depressed, just ok, or on my way to a manic episode. I sort of forget what my normal is. I have suicidal thoughts sometimes, but I call the people closest to me whenever they emerge. I just can't handle another episode. I'm finally doing everything right and I pray that it works long term. My friends and family have all been great and very supportive.

I'm grateful that Hannah saw past my illness and still committed to spend the rest of her life with me. I don't know what I would do without her. I will continue to push forward and hope that someday I can find happiness that doesn't become clinical. The fifth episode set me straight. Now I just have to fend off the sixth.